T0201454

Regression for Health and Social Science

This textbook for students in nontechnical scientific fields covers the basics of linear model methods with a minimum of mathematics, assuming only a precalculus background. Numerous examples drawn from the news and current events, with an emphasis on health issues, illustrate the concepts in an immediately accessible way. Methods covered include linear regression models, Poisson regression, logistic regression, proportional hazards regression, survival analysis, and nonparametric regression.

The author emphasizes interpretation of computer output in terms of the motivating example. All of the **R** code is provided and carefully explained, allowing readers to quickly apply the methods to their own data. Plenty of exercises help students to think about the issues involved in the analysis and its interpretation.

Code and datasets are available for download from the book's website at www .cambridge.org/zelterman

Daniel Zelterman, PhD, is Professor Emeritus, Department of Biostatistics, at Yale University. His application areas include work in clinical trial designs for cancer studies. Before moving to Yale in 1995, he was on the faculty of the University of Minnesota and at the State University of New York at Albany. He is an elected Fellow of the American Statistical Association. In his spare time he plays oboe and bassoon and has backpacked hundreds of miles of the Appalachian Trail.

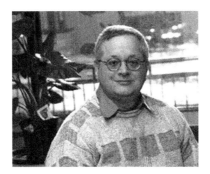

Regression for Health and Social Science

Applied Linear Models with R

DANIEL ZELTERMAN
Yale University, Connecticut

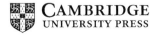

CAMBRIDGE
UNIVERSITY PRESS

CAMBRIDGE
UNIVERSITY PRESS

University Printing House, Cambridge CB2 8BS, United Kingdom

One Liberty Plaza, 20th Floor, New York, NY 10006, USA

477 Williamstown Road, Port Melbourne, VIC 3207, Australia

314–321, 3rd Floor, Plot 3, Splendor Forum, Jasola District Centre,
New Delhi – 110025, India

103 Penang Road, #05–06/07, Visioncrest Commercial, Singapore 238467

Cambridge University Press is part of the University of Cambridge.

It furthers the University's mission by disseminating knowledge in the pursuit of
education, learning, and research at the highest international levels of excellence.

www.cambridge.org
Information on this title: www.cambridge.org/highereducation/isbn/9781108478182
DOI: 10.1017/9781108784504

First published 2022

Printed in the United Kingdom by TJ Books Limited, Padstow, Cornwall, 2022

A catalogue record for this publication is available from the British Library.

ISBN 978-1-108-47818-2 Hardback

Additional resources for this publication at www.cambridge.org/zelterman

Contents

Preface

Linear models are a powerful and useful set of methods in a large number of settings. Briefly, there is some important outcome measurement and we want to explain variations in its values in terms of other measurements in the data. The heights of several trees can be explained in terms of the trees' ages, for example. It is not a straight-line relationship, of course, but knowledge of a tree's age offers us a large amount of explanatory value. We might also want to take into account the effects of measurements on the amount of light, water, nutrients, and weather conditions experienced by each tree. Some of these measurements will have greater explanatory value than others, and we may want to quantify the relative usefulness of these different measures. Even after we are given all of this information, some trees will appear to thrive and others will remain stunted, when all are subjected to identical conditions. Understanding this type of variability is the whole reason for the existence of statistics as a scientific discipline. We usually try to avoid use of the word "prediction" because this assumes there is a cause-and-effect relationship. A tree's age does not directly cause it to grow, for example, but rather, a cumulative process associated with many environmental factors results in increasing height and continued survival. The best estimate we can make is a statement about the behavior of the average tree under identical conditions.

Many of my students go on to work in the pharmaceutical or healthcare industries after graduating with a master's degree. Consequently, the choice of examples in this book has a decidedly health or medical bias. We expect our students to be useful to their employers the day they leave our program, so there is not a lot of time to spend on advanced theory that is not directly applicable. Not all of the examples are from the health sciences. Diverse examples such as the number of lottery winners and temperatures in various US cities are part of our common knowledge. Such examples do not need a lengthy explanation in order for the reader to appreciate many of the aspects of the data being presented.

How is this book different from the many available on the market? The mathematical content and notation are kept to an absolute minimum. To paraphrase the noted physicist Steven Hawking, who wrote extensively for the popular audience, every equation loses half of your audience. There is really no need for formulas and their derivations in a book of this type if we rely on the computer to calculate quantities of interest. Long gone are the days of doing statistics with calculators or on the back of an envelope. Students of mathematical statistics should be able to provide the derivations of the formulas, but they represent a very different audience. All the important formulas are programmed in software so there is no need for the general user to know these.

The three important skills needed by a well-educated student of applied statistics are as follows.

1. Recognize the appropriate method needed in a given setting.
2. Have the necessary computer skills to perform the analysis.
3. Be able to interpret the output and draw conclusions in terms of the original data.

This book gives examples to introduce the reader to a variety of commonly encountered settings and provides guidance through these to complete the three goals. Not all possible situations can be described, of course, but the chosen settings include a broad survey of the types of problems the student of applied statistics is likely to run into.

What do I ask of my readers? We still need to use a lot of mathematical concepts such as the connection between a linear equation and drawing the line on X–Y coordinates. There will be algebra and special functions such as square roots and logarithms. Logarithms, while we are on the subject, are always to the base e (= 2.718...) in this book and not base 10.

We will also need a nodding acquaintance with the concepts of calculus. Many of us took calculus in college a long time ago and have not had much need to use it in the years since. Perhaps we intentionally chose a course of study avoiding abstract mathematics. Even so, calculus represents an important and useful tool. The definitions of the derivative of a function (What does this new function represent?) and integral (What does *this* new function represent?) are required, although we will never actually need to find a derivative or an integral. The necessary refresher to these important concepts is given in Section 1.4.

Also helpful is a previous course in statistics. The reader should be familiar with the mean and standard deviation, normal and binomial distributions, and hypothesis tests in general and the chi-squared and t-tests specifically. These important concepts are reviewed in Chapter 2, but an appreciation of these basic ideas is almost a full course in itself. There is a large reliance on p-values in scientific research, so it is important to know exactly what these represent.

There are a number of excellent general purpose statistical software packages available. We have chosen to illustrate our examples using **R** because of its wide acceptance and use in many industries but especially those of healthcare and pharmaceutical. Most of the examples given here are small, to emphasize interpretation and encourage practice. These data sets could be examined by most software packages. **R**, however, is capable of handling much larger data sets so the skills learned here can easily be used if and when much larger projects are encountered later.

The reader should already have some rudimentary familiarity with running **R** on a computer. This would include using the editor to change the program, submitting the program, retrieving and then printing the output. There are also popular point-and-click approaches to data analysis. While these are quick and acceptable, their ease of use comes with the price of not always being able to repeat the analysis because of the lack of a printed record of the steps taken. Data analysis, then, should be reproducible.

We will review some of the basics of **R** but a little hand-holding will prevent some of the agonizing frustrations frequently occurring when first starting out. Running the computer, and more generally doing the exercises in this book, are a very necessary part of learning statistics. Just as you cannot learn to play the piano simply by reading a book, statistical expertise and the accompanying computer skills can only be obtained by hours of actively using them. Again, much like the piano, the instrument is not damaged by playing a wrong note. Nobody will laugh at you if you try something truly outlandish on the computer either. Perhaps something better will come from a new look at a familiar setting. Similarly, the reader is encouraged to look at the data and try a variety of different ways of looking, plotting, modeling, transforming, and manipulating. Unlike a mathematical problem with only one correct solution (contrary to many of our preconceived notions) there is often a lot of flexibility in the way statistics can be applied to summarize a set of data. As with yet another analogy to music, there are many ways to play the same song.

Acknowledgments

Thanks to the many students and teaching assistants who have provided useful comments and suggestions to the exposition as well as the computer assignments. Also to Beth Nichols, Chang Yu, and Steven Schwager for their careful readings of early drafts of the manuscript. Lauren Cowles and her staff at Cambridge University Press provided innumerable improvements and links to useful websites.

Figure Credits

Figure 1.1: Courtesy of Pennsylvania State University, Department of Meteorology.

Figure 1.4: From the US Census.

Figure 1.5: From Stuckler D, King LP, and Basu S (2008). International Monetary Fund programs and tuberculosis outcomes in post-communist countries. *PLOS Medicine*. Available online at doi:10.1371/journal.pmed.0050143

Figure 1.6: From *The New York Times* (August 15, 2008). © 2008 The New York Times Company. All rights reserved. Used under license.

Figure 1.7: From *The New York Times* (August 4, 2008). © 2008 The New York Times Company. All rights reserved. Used under license.

Figure 1.8: From *The New York Times* (August 23, 2008). © 2008 The New York Times Company. All rights reserved. Used under license.

Figure 1.10: From *The New York Times* (October 14, 2008). © 2008 The New York Times Company. All rights reserved. Used under license.

Table 2.1: From Frisby JP and Clatworthy JL (1975). Learning to see complex random-dot stereograms. *Perception* **4**: 173–8. © Sage Publishing with permission from Pion Ltd.

Figure 2.2: Courtesy of John Huchra.

Table 2.4: On the cognitive penetrability of posture control, N. Teasdale, C. Bard, J. Larue et al., *Experimental Aging Research*, © 1993 Taylor & Francis, reprinted by permission of the publisher (Taylor & Francis Group, www.informaworld.com).

Table 3.1: Data from US Census and used with permission of The Baseball Cube.

Figure 3.4: Prepared by US Drought Monitor, University of Nebraska–Lincoln and updated daily.

Table 3.7: Data obtained from the US National Centers for Environmental Information www.ncdc.noaa.gov and the Florida annual cancer registry www.floridahealth.gov/.

Table 4.5: Data from the World Economic Forum and also appeared in www.reuters .com/article/us-japan-companies-women/women-in-management-at-japan-firms-still-a-rarity-reuters-poll-idUSKCN1LT3GF

Figure 4.5: From the Bureau of Transportation Statistics.

Figures 6.1: reprinted from Cokol M, Chua HN, Tasan M, *et al.* (2011). Systematic exploration of synergistic drug pairs. *Molecular Systems Biology* **7**: Article number 544; /http//doi:10.1038/msb.2011.71

Figures 6.2: Reprinted from Cokol M, Chua HN, Tasan M, *et al.* (2011). Systematic exploration of synergistic drug pairs. *Molecular Systems Biology* **7**: Article number 544; /http//doi:10.1038/msb.2011.71

Table 6.3: Data from the Energy Information Administration.

Table 6.5: Data from the Massachusetts Department of Public Health.

Table 6.7: From Koziol JA, Maxwell DA, Fukushima M, Colmerauer MEM, and Pilch YH (1981). A distribution-free test for tumor-growth curve analysis with application to an animal tumor immunotherapy experiment. *Biometrics* 37: 383–90. Reprinted with permission of Wiley.

Table 7.1: From *Introduction To Generalized Linear Models*, second edition by Dobson AJ. © 2001 by CRC Press. Reproduced with permission of Taylor & Francis Group LLC.

Figure 7.2: From the New York State Education Department.

Table 9.5: Data obtained from the US National Weather Service.

Figure 10.2: From Datagraver.com based on data from the START Global Terrorism Database.

Table 10.6: From van Wattum PJ, Chappell PB, Zelterman D, Scahill LD, and Lecktman JF (2000). Patterns of response to acute Naxolone infusion in Tourette's Syndrome. *Movement Disorders* **15**: 1252–4. Reprinted with permission of Oxford University Press.

Figure 11.2: Wheler J, Tsimberidou AM, Hong D, *et al.* (2009). Survival of patients in a Phase I clinic. *Cancer* **115**(7): 1091–9. © 2009 American Cancer Society.

Table 11.3: From Fleming T, O'Fallon JR, O'Brien PD, and Harrington DP (1980). Modified Kolmogorov–Smirnov test procedures with application to arbitrarily right-censored data. *Biometrics* **36**: 607–25. Reprinted with permission of Wiley.

1 Introduction

We are surrounded by data. With a tap at a computer keyboard, we have access to more than we could possibly absorb in a lifetime. But is this data the same as information? How do we get from numbers to understanding? How do we identify simplifying trends – but also find exceptions to the rule? The computers provide access to the data and also provide the tools to answer these questions. Unfortunately, owning a hammer does not enable us to build a fine house. It takes experience using the tools, knowing when they are appropriate, and also knowing their limitations.

The study of statistics provides the tools to create understanding out of raw data. Expertise comes with experience, of course. We need equal amounts of theory (in the form of statistical tools), technical skills (at the computer), and critical analysis (identifying the limitations of various methods for each setting). A lack of one of these cannot be made up by the other two.

This chapter provides a review of statistics in general, along with the mathematical and statistical prerequisites used in subsequent chapters. More broadly, the reader will be reminded of the larger picture. It is very easy to learn many statistical methods only to lose sight of the point of it all. We will work to provide just enough theory in order to appreciate better the methods provided in subsequent chapters.

1.1 What Is Statistics?

In an effort to present a lot of mathematical formulas, we sometimes lose track of the central idea of the discipline. It is important to remember the big picture when we get too close to the subject.

Let us consider a vast wall separating our lives from the place where the information resides. It is impossible to see over or around this wall, but every now and then we have the good fortune of having some pieces of data thrown over to us. On the basis of this fragmentary sampled data, we need to infer the composition of the remainder on the other side. This is the aim of *statistical inference*. The population is usually vast and infinite, whereas the sample is just a handful of numbers.

> In statistical inference we infer properties
> of the population from the sample.

There is an enormous possibility for error, of course. If all of the left-handed people I know also have artistic ability, am I allowed to generalize this to conclude all left-handed people are artistic? I may not know very many left-handed people. In this case I do not have much data to make my claim and my statement should reflect a large possibility of error. Maybe most of my friends are also artists. In this case we say the sampled data is *biased* because it contains more artists than would be found in a representative sample of the population.

The population in this example is the totality of all left-handed people. Maybe the population should be *all* people, if we also want to show artistic ability is greater in left-handed people than in right-handed people. We can't possibly measure such a large group. Instead, we must resign ourselves to the observed or *empirical* data made up of the people we know. This is called a *convenience sample* because it is not really random and may not be representative.

Consider next the separate concepts of sample and population for numerically valued data. The sample *average* is a number we use to infer the value of the population *mean*. The average of several numbers is itself a number we obtain. The population mean, however, is on the other side of the imaginary wall and is not observable. The population mean is almost an unknowable quantity, unobservable even after a lifetime of study. Fortunately, statistical inference allows us to make statements about the population mean on the basis of the sample average. Sometimes we forget inference is taking place and confuse the sample statistic with the population attribute.

Statistics are functions of the sampled data.
Parameters are properties of the population.

Often the sampled data comes at great expense and through personal hardship, as in the case of clinical trials of new therapies for life-threatening diseases. In a clinical trial in cancer, for example, costs are typically many thousands of dollars per patient enrolled. Innovative therapies can easily cost much more. Sometimes the most important data consists of a single number, such as how long the patient lived, recorded only after the patient loses the fight with their disease.

Sometimes we attempt to collect all of the data, as in the case of a *census*. The US Constitution specifically mandates a complete census of the population be performed every 10 years.[1] The writers of the Constitution knew that, in order to have a representative democracy and a fair tax system, we also need to know where the people live and work. The composition of the House of Representatives is based on the decennial census. Locally, communities need to know about population shifts to plan for schools and roads. Despite the importance of the census data, there continues to be

---

[1] Article 1, Section 2 reads, in part: "Representatives and direct Taxes shall be apportioned among the several States which may be included within this Union, according to their respective Numbers, which shall be determined by adding to the whole Number of free Persons, including those bound to Service for a Term of Years, and excluding Indians not taxed, three fifths of all other Persons. The actual Enumeration shall be made within three Years after the first Meeting of the Congress of the United States, and within every subsequent Term of ten Years, in such Manner as they shall by Law direct."

controversy on how to identify and count certain segments of the population, including the homeless, prison inmates, migrant workers, college students, and foreign persons living in the country without appropriate documentation. For most of our work, a census is out of the question. Instead, we must rely on a *sample* and then generalize from a sample of data to the larger population.

The sample average is a simple statistic immediately coming to mind. The Student t-test is the principal method used to make inference about the population mean on the basis of the sample average. We review this method in Section 2.5. The sample *median* is the value at which half of the sample is above and half is below. The median is discussed in Chapter 7. We next discuss statistical measures of variability.

> The standard deviation measures how far individual
> observations deviate from their average.

The sample *standard deviation* allows us to estimate the scale or variability in the population. On the basis of the normal distribution (Section 2.3), we usually expect about 68% of the population to appear within one standard deviation (above or below) of the mean. Similarly, about 95% of the population should occur within two standard deviations of the population mean.

> The standard error measures the sampling variability of the mean.

A commonly used measure related to the standard deviation is the *standard error*, also called the *standard error of the mean* and often abbreviated SEM. These two similar-sounding quantities refer to very different measures.

The standard error estimates the variability associated with the sample average. As the sample size increases, the standard deviation (which refers to individuals in the population) should not appreciably change. On the other hand, a large sample size is associated with a precise estimate of the population mean. As a consequence, a small standard error is a result of a large sample. This relationship provides the incentive for larger sample sizes, allowing us to estimate the population mean more accurately.

The relationship is as follows.

$$\text{Standard error} = \frac{\text{Standard deviation}}{\sqrt{\text{Sample size}}}$$

Consider a simple example. We want to measure the heights of a group of people. There will always be tall people, and there will always be short people, so changing the sample size does not appreciably alter the standard deviation of the data. Individual variations will always be observed. If we are interested in estimating the average height, then the standard error will decrease with an increase in the sample size (at a rate of $1/\sqrt{\text{sample size}}$), motivating the use of ever-larger samples. The average will be measured with greater precision, and this precision is described in terms of the standard error. Similarly, if we want to measure the average with twice the precision, then we will need a sample size four times larger.

Another commonly used term associated with the standard deviation is *variance*. The relationship between the variance and the standard deviation is as follows.

$$\text{Variance} = (\text{Standard deviation})^2$$

The standard deviation and variance are obtained in **R** using sd() and var() functions. The formula appears often and the reader should be familiar with it, even though its value will be calculated using a computer.

Given observed sample values $x_1, x_2, \ldots, x_n$, we compute the *sample variance* from

$$s^2 = \text{sample variance} = \frac{1}{n-1} \sum_i (x_i - \bar{x})^2, \tag{1.1}$$

where $\bar{x}$ is the average of the observed values.

This estimate is often denoted by the symbol s^2. Similarly, the estimated sample standard deviation s is the square root of this estimator. Intuitively, we see that (1.1) averages the squared difference between each observation and the sample average, except the denominator is one less than the sample size. The "$n-1$" term counts the degrees of freedom for this expression and is described in Sections 2.5 and 2.7.

1.2   Statistics in the News: the Weather Map

Sometimes it is possible to be overwhelmed with too much information. The business news is filled with stock prices, and the sports section has a similar wealth of scores and data on athletic endeavors. The business news frequently has several graphs and charts illustrating trends, rates, and prices. Sports writers have yet to catch up with business reporters in terms of these types of aids for the reader.

As an excellent way to summarize and display a huge amount of information, we reproduce the US weather map in Fig. 1.1 for an autumn day. There are several levels of information depicted here, all overlaid one on top of another. First we recognize the geographic–political map indicating the shorelines and state boundaries. The large map, Fig. 1.1 (a), provides the details of the day's weather. The large Hs indicate the locations of high-barometric-pressure centers. Regions with similar temperatures are displayed in the same colors. The locations of rain and snow are indicated. An element of time and movement can also be inferred from this map: A large front has come across the country from the north, bringing cooler temperatures along with it. This figure represents the fine art of summarizing a huge amount of information.

The two smaller maps, Figs. 1.1 (b) and (c), provide a different kind of information. Map (b) indicates the temperatures we should expect at this time of year, based on previous years' experiences. The general pattern follows our preconception that southern

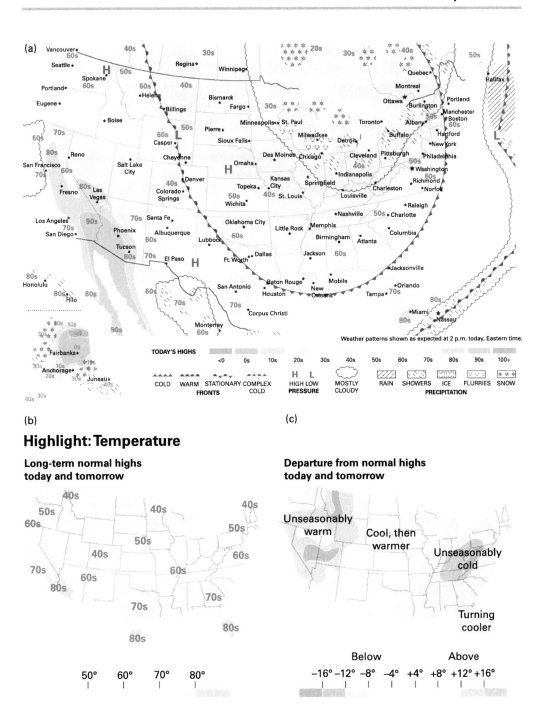

Figure 1.1 The US weather map: (a) observed, (b) expected, and (c) residual data. Courtesy of Pennsylvania State University, Department of Meteorology.

states are warmer and northern states are cooler at this time of the year, with bands of constant temperature running east and west.

Map (c) summarizes the differences between the normal pattern and the temperatures given in map (a). Here we see Florida is usually warm but much cooler than expected for late autumn. Similarly, Montana is normally cold at this time of year but is much warmer than typical.

The aim of statistics is to provide a similar reduction of a large amount of data into a succinct statement, generalizing, summarizing, and providing a clear message to your audience.

> An important goal of statistics is to prepare a concise summary of the data.

1.3   Mathematical Background

Many of us chose to study health or social sciences and shunned engineering or physics in order to avoid the abstract rigor of mathematics. However, much of the research in the social and health fields is quantitative. We still need to demonstrate the benefit of any proposed intervention or social observation in numerical terms.

For example, we all know the role the American Society for the Prevention of Cruelty to Animals (ASPCA) and other animal shelters perform in protecting homeless cats and dogs. It only takes a quick visit to their local facilities to assess the effectiveness of their efforts. We can easily count the number of charges under their care to quantify and measure what they do. In this example it is easy to separate the emotional appeal from the quantity of good such an organization supplies.

In contrast, we are shocked to see the brutality of whales being slaughtered. We are told about the majesty of their huge size and life under the sea. This is all fine but also plays on our emotions. Before we send money to fund the appropriate charity, or decide to enforce global bans on whaling, we also should ask how many whales there are, and perhaps how this number has changed over the past decade.

This information is much harder to get at and is outside our day-to-day experiences. We need to rely on estimates to quantify the problem. Perhaps we also need to question who is providing these estimates and whether the estimates are biased to support a certain point of view. An objective estimate of the whale population may be difficult to obtain, yet it is crucial to quantifying the problem.

As a consequence, we need to use some level of mathematics to help with our task. Of course, much of mathematics is an abstract, oversimplification of what is really happening. But it is through this simplification, we can learn, turning data into understanding the overall trend. Notice how the map in Fig. 1.1 (a) is simplified by the two maps in Figs. 1.1 (b) and (c).

The computer will do most of the heavy lifting for us, but we will still need to understand what is going on behind the scenes. We need to use algebra and especially linear functions. So when we write

$$y = a + bx,$$

recall a is referred to as the *intercept* and b is called the *slope*. We need to recognize this equation represents a straight-line relationship and be able to graph this relationship.

We will need to use logarithms. Logarithms, or logs for short, are always to the base e $= 2.718\ldots$ and never to base 10 in this book.

The exponential function written as e^x or $\exp(x)$ is the inverse process of the logarithm. That is,

$$\log(e^x) = x$$

and

$$e^{\log x} = \exp(\log x) = x.$$

Sometimes we will use the exponential notation when the argument is not a simple expression. Otherwise, we write exp() instead of "e to the power."

1.4   Calculus

For those who took calculus a long time ago and have not used it since, the memories may be distant and perhaps unpleasant. Calculus represents a collection of important mathematical tools needed from time to time in our discussion later on in this book. We will need to use several useful results requiring calculus.

Fortunately, there is no need to dig out and dust off long-forgotten textbooks. The actual mechanics of calculus will be reviewed here, but there will not be a need actually to perform the mathematics involved. The reader who is fluent in the relevant mathematics may be able to fill in the details we will gloss over.

What is the point of calculus? If x and y have a straight-line relationship, we should be familiar with the concept of the *slope* of the line. When x changes by one unit, the slope is the amount of change in y.

For a nonlinear relationship, the concept of the slope remains the same but it is a more local phenomenon. The idea of the slope depends on where in the x–y relationship our interest lies. At any point in a curve, we can still talk about the slope, but we need to talk about the slope at each point of the curve. You might think of a curve as a lot of tiny linear segments all sewn together, end to end. In this case, the concept of slope is the ratio of a small change in y to the small change in x at a given point on the curve. It still makes sense to talk about the ratio of these small amounts resulting in a definition of the slope of a curved line at every point x. In calculus, the *derivative* is a measure of the (local) slope at any given point in the function.

The derivative of a function provides its slope at each point.

(a)   (b)

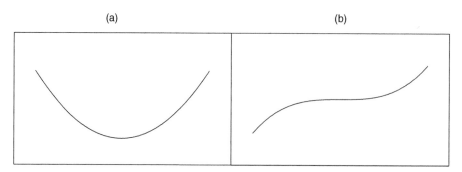

Figure 1.2 The slope is zero at the minimum of a function (a) and also at the saddle point of a function (b).

The derivative is useful for identifying places where nonlinear functions achieve their minimums or maximums. Intuitively, we can see a smooth function decreasing for a while and then increasing so it will have to pass through a point where the slope is zero. Solving for the places where the derivative is zero tells us where the original function is either maximized or minimized. See Fig. 1.2 (a) for an illustration of this concept.

Some functions also exhibit *saddle points* where the derivative is zero. A saddle point is where an increasing function flattens out before resuming its increase. A saddle point is illustrated in Fig. 1.2 (b). We will not concern ourselves with saddle points. Similarly, a zero value of the derivative may only indicate a local minimum or maximum (that is, there are either larger maximums or smaller minimums somewhere else), but we will not be concerned with these topics either.

Although we will not actually obtain derivatives in this book, on occasion we will need to minimize and maximize functions. When the need arises, we will recognize the need to take a derivative and set it to zero and solve in order to identify where the minimum occurs.

> The derivative is zero where the smooth function
> achieves a maximum or minimum.

Calculus is also concerned with *integrals of functions*. Briefly, an integral gives us the area between the function and the horizontal axis. As with the derivative, we will not actually need to derive one here. Many probabilities are determined according to the area under a curved function and these can be found easily in **R**.

> The integral of a function provides the area between
> the curve and the horizontal x axis.

Specifically, when we examine the normal distribution (Section 2.3), we will often draw the familiar bell-shaped curve. This curve is illustrated in Fig. 1.3. For any value x on the horizontal axis, curve (b) gives us the cumulative area under curve

(a)   (b)

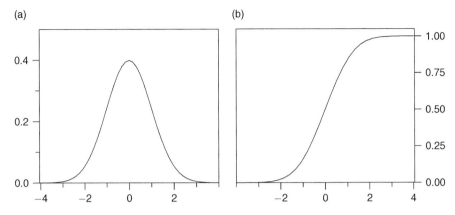

Figure 1.3 The normal density function (a) and its cumulative area (b).

(a), up to x. The total area on part (a) is 1, and the cumulative area increases up to this value.

The cumulative area under this curve is almost always of greater interest to us than the bell curve itself. It is very rare to see a table of the bell curve. Both the bell curve and its integral are easily found in **R**. This will be illustrated in Section 2.3.

The area can be negative if the function has a negative value. Negative areas may seem unintuitive, but the example in Section 1.5 illustrates this concept.

1.5 Calculus in the News: New-Home Construction

Building starts for new homes are an important part of the economy. Builders will not start an expensive project unless they are reasonably sure their investment will pay off. Home buyers will usually purchase new furniture and carpets, and hire painters and carpenters to remodel as they move in. Investors, economists, and government policy makers watch this data as a sign of the current state of the economy as well as future trends.

The graphs in Fig. 1.4 are based on US Census data up to the middle of 2018. There are always new homes being built and put up for sale, of course, but it is useful to know whether the trend is increasing or decreasing. Figure 1.4 (b) shows the trend in terms of the annual changes. More specifically, graph (b) approximates the slope of the line in graph (a) at the corresponding point in time. When the graph (a) is increasing, then graph (b) is positive. Decreasing rates in (a) correspond to negative values in (b).

In words, graph (b) is the derivative of graph (a). Similarly, if we start at the values corresponding to the start of the year 1990, then graph (a) is obtained by integrating the values in graph (b). Areas under the negative values in (b) integrate to "negative areas" so the negative values in (b) correspond to declining values in (a).

The times at which the derivatives in (b) are zero correspond to turning points where maximums or minimums occur in (a). Remember a zero slope is usually indicative

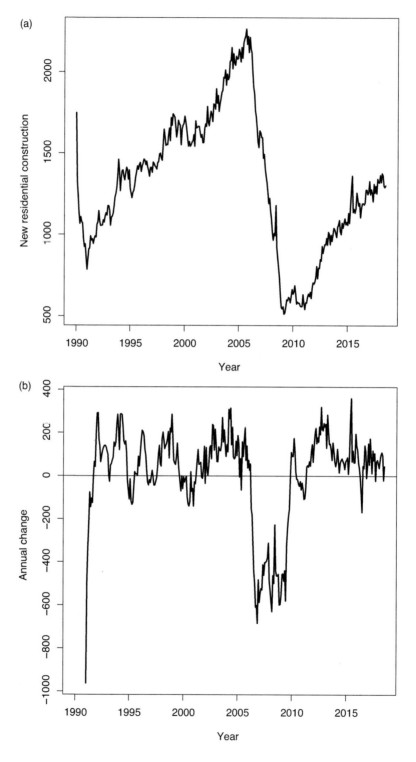

Figure 1.4 (a) New residential construction starts and (b) annual change.
Source: US Census.

of a change in direction. These maximums or minimums may be short-lived, of course, and the underlying trend may continue after they end. The wide swings in the derivative often allow us to anticipate a change in direction of the underlying trend by a few months.

The large decline in the economy in 2008 corresponded to a large drop in housing starts. Similarly, the annual change at that time was a large negative number. A large jump in the annual change seemed to signal a change in the trend and homes were once again being built at a prerecession rate in 2010.

What do these two graphs tell us about the near future in home building, and the economy, more generally? Exercise 1.1a sks you to argue both cases: in the near term the economy is improving; and also, the economy is getting worse.

1.6   A Cautionary Tale

It is possible to learn about statistics, computing, and data analysis and still come to an absurd conclusion. This sometimes leads to sensational headlines with often hilarious results as the story unfolds.

Figure 1.5 is reprinted from an article by Stuckler *et al.* (2008). A summary of the original article appeared in the *New York Times* on July 22, 2008.[2]

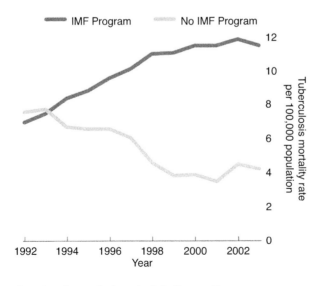

Figure 1.5 Cases of tuberculosis in Eastern Europe.
Source: Stuckler *et al.* (2008).

---

[2] The original article is available online from *PLOS Medicine*: https://doi.org/10.1371/journal.pmed .0050143. A critique of this article appears at https://doi.org/10.1371/journal.pmed.0050162

The article is about the relationship between International Monetary Fund (IMF) loans and the rate of tuberculosis (TB) in various eastern European countries. TB is an infectious disease spread through the air when an affected person sneezes or coughs. The disease is treated using antibiotics and is frequently fatal if left untreated. The elderly, those with diabetes, and those with a weakened immune system (such as those with human immunodeficiency virus or HIV) are at high risk for TB. We frequently see cases of TB in crowded living conditions with poor sanitation.

The IMF (www.imf.org) is an international organization overseeing the global monetary system, including exchange rates, balance of payments, and sometimes making loans to foreign governments. Critics of the IMF claim the conditions imposed on these loans will cause more harm than good to the population. These conditions have included forcing a nation to raise taxes or increase exports to the exclusion of food production needed at home. Critics will be able to point to this graph and claim the IMF conditions result in cuts in preventive public health expenditures and reductions in the availability of necessary vaccines. Imposing these conditions on the recipient nations has resulted in crowded and unsanitary living conditions, thereby raising the incidence of TB.

In the original article, the authors performed a large number of statistical analyses to take into account differences in the various countries with respect to percent of the population living in urban settings, an index of democratization, differences in per-capita incomes, whether or not the country was involved in a war, and population education levels. Most of the methods used in their article will be clear to the reader by the time we complete the material in Chapter 6.

Even so, not all countries are the same. There may be large differences between the countries these analyses fail to correct for. Are there other factors not taken into account? Could factors such as the age of the population or the rates of HIV infection result in the differences in TB rates, regardless of whether or not the nation received IMF loans?

How should we treat countries applying for IMF loans but not qualifying? Should these be considered loan recipients? Similarly, some countries may have been offered loans but ultimately refused the money. Should these countries be considered as having received loans? What about the size of the loans? Would a large loan have the same effect as a small loan if few conditions were attached to it?

Even more importantly, this is an example of an *observational study*. Why did some countries receive loans while others did not? In what ways do these countries differ? We will never be able to know the effect on TB rates if a given country not receiving a loan had been given one, or vice versa. Consider Exercise 1.2 for another possible interpretation of Fig. 1.5. In an observational study, the subjects (in this case, individual countries) choose their causal treatment in some nonrandom fashion. In the present example, we do not know how countries were chosen to receive loans.

We could not randomly choose the countries to receive loans. A *randomized study*, in contrast to an observational study, allows us randomly to assign treatments to individuals. Differences in outcomes can then be attributed solely to the random assignment. In a medical study in which patients are randomly assigned to two different treatments, for example, any underlying imbalances in the two patient-group outcomes should be minimized by chance alone. Patients bearing a trait unknown to us at the time of the randomization would be equally likely to appear in either of the two treatment groups and then the trait would be averaged out when we examine the outcome. However, it is not possible randomly to give or withhold IMF loans to the various countries in the study.

One final comment on this example: Why was TB chosen to illustrate the effects of IMF loans? Of all the various disease rates reported, what is special about TB? Is it possible the authors studied many different disease rates, but only TB proved to be the most remarkable? We don't know how many diseases were compared between IMF loan and nonloan nations. Clearly, if many comparisons were made then it is virtually certain some remarkable findings will be uncovered. One disease rate out of many must appear to have the largest difference between loan and nonloan nations.

This is the problem with *multiple comparisons*. If many comparisons are made, then the largest of these is not representative. We would need to make a correction for the number of different diseases studied. This topic and an appropriate adjustment for multiple comparisons are discussed again in Section 2.4.

There are many lessons we can learn from this example. Ultimately, a study of statistical methods will provide you with a very useful set of tools. This book shows how these can be used to gain insight into underlying trends and patterns in your data. These tools, however, are only as good as your data.

Of course, if you also abuse the methods, it is possible to do more damage than good. You may be using the most sophisticated statistical methods available, but you are still responsible for your final conclusions. An extreme example is presented in Section 4.5.4 where four very different sets of data give rise to the same summary values.

Statistics is a useful tool, but it cannot think for you.

The same advice also holds for computers. Software can churn out numbers, but it cannot tell you whether the methods are appropriate or if the conditions for these methods are valid. For other examples of statistics in action, consider the exercises at the end of this chapter. As with every chapter in this book, work out as many as you can.

1.7   Exercises

1.1   How could we use the data in Fig. 1.4 to argue the economy is improving? Use the same data and discuss how this shows the economy is in decline. Would it be useful to look at the derivative of graph (b), that is, the second derivative of graph (a), in order to judge a change in the direction of the trend? We could estimate this by looking at the changes from the previous years' values in graph (b).

1.2 Can we make the case a country with a high rate of TB is more likely to receive an IMF loan? That is to say, use Fig. 1.5 to claim TB causes loans, rather than the other way around.

1.3 Do cell phones cause brain cancer? Does extensive use of a cell phone constitute a randomized experiment or an observational study? Describe the person who is most likely to be a big user of their cell phone. Is this a fair cross-section of the population?

1.4 Several US states have passed laws to stop drivers from using cell phones. Do cell phones cause traffic accidents? Are people who own cell phones, but don't use them while driving, more likely to be involved in accidents?

1.5 Does consumption of soft drinks cause conjunctivitis (pink eye)? Cases of pink eye occur most often during the same months in which soft drink consumption is greatest. What do you think is going on?

1.6 A study found higher rates of obesity among ninth graders whose school is located close to a fast-food outlet.[3] In another part of the same study, pregnant women who lived near a fast-food outlet were more likely to experience a huge gain in weight. Are these experiments or observations? See if you can provide several different explanations for these findings.

1.7.1 Motorcycle Accidents

In Fig. 1.6 (a) we see the number of motor vehicle fatalities has held steady over the two decades 1987–2007.[4] The right-hand graph in part (a) shows the number of fatalities per miles traveled is declining. Which of these two graphs is a better indication of highway safety? Is there additional information you would need before making this conclusion? Are all travel miles the same, for example? Are there more or fewer cars on the road? Are the drivers younger or older, on average?

The two graphs in Fig. 1.6 (b) indicate there has been a recent increase in fatalities involving motorcycles and these make up an increasing percentage of all accident fatalities. What additional information would you like to see? Use this graph to show how inherently dangerous motorcycles are. In contrast, use this graph and argue motorcycles are as safe as other motor vehicles. We can use the same data to make a case for both sides of this debate.

1.7.2 Olympic Records

In the modern history of the Olympics, we accumulate records as the athletes are running faster than ever before. Figure 1.7 plots the times of various track events, separately for men (a) and women (b). In order to make these different events comparable, the average pace speeds are plotted as the time to cover 100 m. Speeds are faster

---

[3] Available online at www.nytimes.com/2009/03/26/health/nutrition/26obese.html.
[4] Available online at www.nytimes.com/2008/08/15/us/15fatal.html.

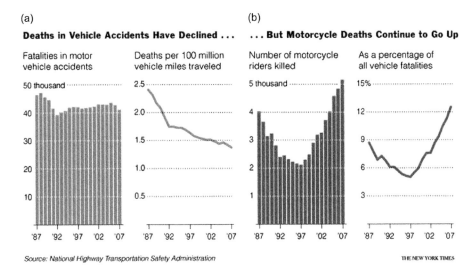

(a)

Deaths in Vehicle Accidents Have Declined . . .

Fatalities in motor vehicle accidents

Deaths per 100 million vehicle miles traveled

(b)

. . . But Motorcycle Deaths Continue to Go Up

Number of motorcycle riders killed

As a percentage of all vehicle fatalities

Source: National Highway Transportation Safety Administration

THE NEW YORK TIMES

Figure 1.6 Fatality rates for (a) autos and (b) motorcycles. Source: *New York Times*, August 15, 2008, page A11.

from top to bottom. Shorter distances are bursts of energy and are much faster than the marathon (26+ miles), in which runners need to hold back and conserve their strength for the long haul. Similarly, the slower marathon times appear at the top, and shorter sprints are given at the bottom. Earlier data was timed using a hand-held stopwatch, which was less accurate than the electronic methods used in today's Olympics.

Which events seem to have attained a plateau and only small improvements are appearing? Similarly, which events continue to be run faster than ever before? Which events are most likely to produce new records at the next Olympics? Which of these will represent large improvements over the previous records? Would you rather see a record representing a small improvement of a fraction of a second over previous speeds or a large jump in a record time continuing to hold for decades? Which type of record would generate the greatest excitement for present or subsequent Olympics?

Consider the slope and intercept for the various lines in this figure. Specifically, compare the slope and intercept of the marathon rates for men and women. Which line has the larger intercept? Which has the larger slope? The women's record times are slower, and this line is higher than the men's. Which of these lines is steeper? Why is this the case? Does it appear there will be a time when women run faster marathons than men? How far into the future might this occur? There is a danger in extrapolating beyond the observed data. This cannot be overemphasized.

1.7.3   Gasoline Consumption

Figure 1.8 presents graphs of gasoline price, consumption, and miles driven in the United States. We see a general trend of fewer miles driven in graph (a). Or do we? The numbers being plotted are all positive, except for the most recent data and a brief

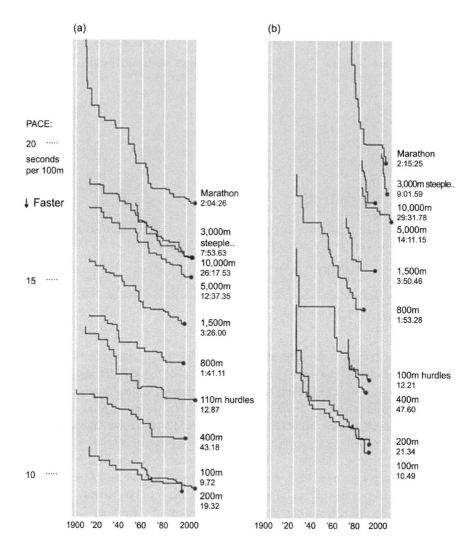

Figure 1.7 Olympic records for men's track events (a) and women's track events (b) in the twentieth century. Source: *New York Times*, August 4, 2008.

period in 1990. Look again: Are fewer miles being driven? In terms of calculus, are we looking at the number of miles driven, or its derivative?

Notice the different time scales involved. We see a trend of prices of gasoline increasing and less being purchased from June 2008 to August 2008. The graph of prices (c) is much smoother than either of the other two figures. Why is this the case? During this period, the price of gasoline roughly trended in the opposite direction from the gasoline-purchased graph (b). A $600 per person economic stimulus check was distributed during this period, as indicated by the shaded areas. Did this appear to have any effect?

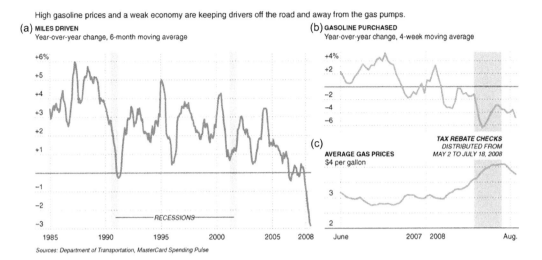

High gasoline prices and a weak economy are keeping drivers off the road and away from the gas pumps.

Figure 1.8 Gasoline consumption and prices. Source: *New York Times*, August 23, 2008, Page C3.

1.7.4 Foreign Owners of US Treasury Debt

Much of the US debt issued by the Treasury has been purchased by foreign governments, institutions, and individuals. As the United States of America imports foreign products, US dollars make their way overseas. These make their way back to the USA in the form of investments and purchases of debt in the form of bonds. The purchases are made by governments, and large institutions such as foreign banks, pension funds, and insurance companies. There may also be undisclosed sources, such as those investments made though Luxembourg.

In the years leading up to the time period covered by the graph shown in Fig. 1.9, there was a lot of talk about a great trade imbalance between the USA and China leading to tariffs and fees levied on imported goods. From Fig. 1.9, what can you say about the resulting investment in Treasury bonds by China? Similarly, there has been a large increase in bond ownership in Japan. There is a large amount of variability within the year, specially in Japan and the UK.

Also, the dollars are undergoing inflation, and earlier years' dollars are worth more than recent dollars. At the time the graph in Fig. 1.9 appeared, interest rates returned on bonds were very low, so investors may have received less return on their money. Perhaps this information is useful because there would be less incentive to buy bonds for investment purposes. Maybe the Treasury bonds were purchased for other reasons, such as safety and stability. Does this explain the large holdings from Luxembourg, where the true owners' identities are hidden?

1.7.5 US Presidents and Stock Market Returns

In the 80 years following the great stock market crash of 1929, Democratic and Republican administrations have had almost the same number of years in the White

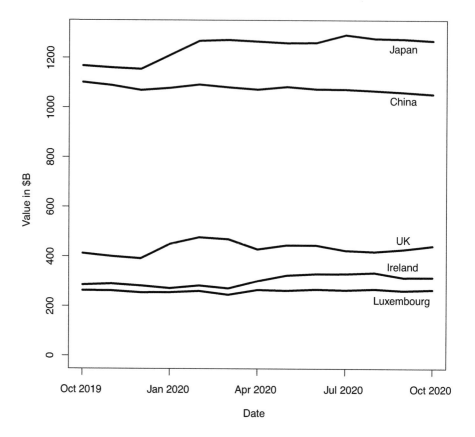

Figure 1.9 Largest foreign owners of US Treasury debt. Source: US Treasury

House: six Democrat and seven Republican US presidents have served almost exactly 40 years each. How well have investors fared under each of these political parties? The average annual return under each president is given in Fig. 1.10 as of mid October, 2008, and we are invited to make this comparison. The figure also provides the data on a hypothetical $10,000 investment made under either Democratic or Republican presidents only.

The Hoover administration was clearly a disaster for investors, losing more than 30% per year on average. Such exceptional observations are called *outliers*. If we average the returns from all of the Republican presidential terms, the result is a meager 0.4% return per year. The $10,000 investment would have grown to $11,733 over this period of 40 years. If we exclude the Hoover years, then the Republican average is 4.7%, resulting in a return of $51,211 after 36 years. Under Democratic presidents, the average return is 8.9% per year, and the $10,000 investment would have become more than $300,000 over 40 years. The figure asks us to conclude investors experience greater rewards under Democratic presidents than under Republican presidents. But is this really the case?

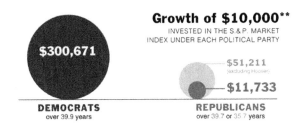

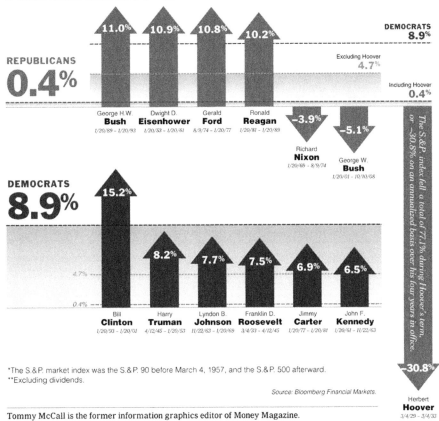

Figure 1.10 Democratic and Republican US presidents and the corresponding returns in the stock market, 1929–2008. Source: *New York Times*, October 14, 2008.

It is clear the returns under President Hoover were out of the ordinary; it also appears only President Clinton's returns were above the Democratic average. That is, as much as Hoover's time in office was an exception on the downside, Clinton's appears to be an exception on the upside.

One way to take exceptional observations into account is to examine the *median* value for each of the two political parties. (When we calculate the median for an even number of observations, as with the Democratic party, we average the two middle values.) What are the median annual returns for each of the two political parties, including the data from President Hoover? Do these lead us to the same conclusion as taking the average? Which of these two statistics do you feel is more representative for these data: the average or the median?

Recognize there is a lot more we could do in order to make a better comparison of the political parties. For example, an average of several different rates over different numbers of years is not the same as a constant rate over those same years. Dividends are not included in the figures. Dividends are income paid by companies to investors who hold their stock and dividends are a part of the return investors will earn as a reward for taking the risk of owning the stock. Dividend rates are tied to current interest rates and may vary with the rate of inflation at the time.

2 Principles of Statistics

There is really no shortcut to taking a full introductory course to cover the basic concepts of statistics. In this chapter we will cover the most important ideas with which the reader should be familiar. Think of this material as a brief refresher to old ideas rather than the true exposure to new topics.

Historically, the development of probability predates the use of statistics by several centuries. The need for probability came about in studies of games of chance. Gamblers were then, as they are today, seeking an edge in an easy way to make a fortune. Of course, if there was a way to do so, there would be many wealthy mathematicians today. Instead, mathematicians have shown there is no winning strategy. Card-counting at blackjack requires considerable practice and great concentration, and only then does it provide a slight edge to the player.

Statistics, on the other hand, was very much a product of the industrial revolution. Large numbers of items needed to be produced in a uniform fashion, and random variability stood in the way. Statistics became a scientific discipline in the early 1900s with the development of two important innovations: the chi-squared test thanks to K. Pearson,[1] and Student's t-test. Both of these topics are reviewed later in this chapter.

2.1 The Binomial Distribution

The binomial distribution is one of the basic mathematical models for describing the behavior of a random outcome. An experiment is performed resulting in one of two complementary outcomes, usually referred to as success and failure. Each experimental outcome occurs independently of the others, and every experiment has the same probability of failure or success.

A toss of a coin is a good example. The coin tosses are independent of each other and the probability of heads or tails is constant from one toss to another. The coin is said to be *fair* if there is an equal probability of heads and tails on each toss. A *biased* coin will favor one outcome over the other. If I toss a coin (whether fair or biased) several times, can I anticipate the numbers of head and tails to be expected? There is no way of knowing with certainty, of course, but some outcomes will be more likely

---

[1] Karl Pearson (1857–1936), British mathematician and biostatistician.

than others. The binomial distribution allows us to calculate a probability for every possible outcome.

Consider another example. Suppose I know from experience when driving through a certain intersection, I will have to stop for the traffic light 80% of the time. Each time I pass, whether or not I have to stop is independent of all of the previous times. The 80% rate never varies. It does not depend on the time of day, the direction I am traveling, nor the amount of traffic on the road. If I pass through this same intersection eight times in one week, the binomial distribution allows me to answer how many times I should expect to have to stop for the light. Similarly, I can ask what is the probability I will have to stop exactly six times in the eight times I pass this intersection?

The binomial model is a convenient mathematical tool to help explain these types of experiences. Let us introduce some notation. Suppose there are N independent events, where N takes on a positive integer value $1, 2, \ldots$. Each experiment either results in a success with probability p or else results in a failure with probability $1 - p$ for some value of p between 0 and 1.

> The binomial distribution provides the probability of the
> number of successes in N independent trials, each
> with the same probability p of success.

Let X denote the number of successes in N trials. The probability X takes on the value i is

$$\Pr[X = i] = \binom{N}{i} p^i (1 - p)^{N-i} \tag{2.1}$$

for any value of $i = 0, 1, \ldots, N$.

We look at the formula for this probability and should think of it as the product of three terms. There are i independent successes, occurring with probability p^i. There are also $N - i$ independent failures with probability $(1 - p)^{N-i}$. Finally, we need to consider all the different ordered ways the various successes and failures could have occurred.

If we look carefully at the formula in (2.1), we see it does not matter which event we call the "success" and which "failure." This equation provides the probability of i outcomes, each occurring with probability p. We could just as well have described the probability of $N - i$ outcomes, each occurring with the probability $1 - p$. Similarly, we can drop the words *success* and *failure* and just say there were i appearances of one event, and $N - i$ appearances of the complementary event.

Recall the factorial symbol (!) is shorthand for the product of all positive integers up to that point. So we have

$$4! = 4 \times 3 \times 2 \times 1 = 24,$$

for example. (We read 4! as "four factorial.")

The binomial coefficient

$$\binom{N}{i} = \frac{N!}{i!\,(N-i)!}$$

counts all the different ordered ways in which i of the N individual experiments could have occurred. (We read this symbol as "N choose i.")

For example, $X = 2$ heads in $N = 4$ tosses of a coin could have occurred as HHTT, HTHT, HTTH, THHT, THTH, or TTHH. The six possible orders in which these occur is also obtained as

$$\binom{4}{2} = \frac{4!}{2!\,2!} = 6.$$

In **R** we can use the `factorial` and `choose` functions.

```
> factorial(4)
[1] 24
> choose(4, 2)
[1] 6
```

A plot of the probabilities in (2.1) is given in Fig. 2.1 for $N = 10$, values of $p = 0.2, 0.5,$ and 0.8, and all values of $i = 0, 1, \ldots, 10$. When $p = 0.2$ we see the distribution favors smaller numbers of events, so observing seven or more successes is very unlikely. When $p = 0.8$ we see a "mirror image," and three or fewer success are rarely expected to occur. The model with $p = 0.5$ in the center is symmetric.

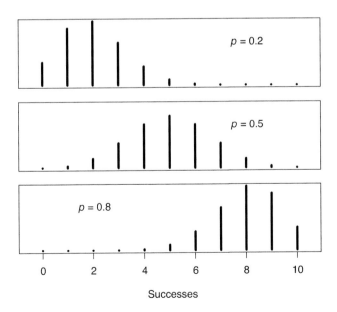

Figure 2.1 The binomial distribution of the number of successes, illustrated for index $N = 10$. The lengths of the vertical lines are the probabilities of each possible outcome.

This symmetric shape is beginning to look like a normal or bell curve. The normal distribution is discussed in Section 2.3.

> When N is large and p is not too close to either 0 or 1, then the binomial model is approximated by the normal distribution.

Returning to the example of eight trips past the intersection, the probability I have to stop six times is

$$\Pr[\, X = 6 \,] = \binom{8}{6} (0.8)^6 (0.2)^2 = 28 \times 0.0105 = 0.2936.$$

The probability I have to stop six or more times is

$$\Pr[\, X \geq 6 \,] = \Pr[\, X = 6 \,] + \Pr[\, X = 7 \,] + \Pr[\, X = 8 \,].$$

These three probabilities need to be evaluated separately using (2.1) and can be found in **R** using the dbinom function to calculate binomial probabilities

```
> dbinom(6 : 8, size = 8, prob = 0.8)
[1] 0.2936013 0.3355443 0.1677722
> sum(dbinom(6 : 8, size = 8, prob = 0.8))
[1] 0.7969178
```

separately finding the individual probabilities and then their sum. Another example is given in Exercise 2.1.

We can also use the dbinom function in **R** to draw the pictures in Fig. 2.1. This script will produce the first of the three plots in this figure.

```
N <- 10
p <- 0.2
plot(c(0, N), c(0, .4), type = "n",
     ylab = "Probability", xlab = "Number of successes")
for (i in 0:N)
    lines(rep(i,2), c(0, dbinom(i,N,p)), type = "l", lwd = 3)
```

The plot statement specifies the limits of the figure. The type = "n" specifies no plotting, producing only an empty frame and labels on the a margins. The lines statements produces a separate line each individual probability.

Returning to properties of the binomial distribution, the expected number of successes is

$$\text{Expected number of successes} = Np \qquad (2.2)$$

and the variance of the number of successes is

$$\text{Variance of the number of successes} = Np(1 - p). \qquad (2.3)$$

> The binomial distribution has expected value Np
> and variance $Np(1 - p)$.

Intuitively, the mean number of successes is Np. The variance of the number of successes is also the variance of the number of failures. The variance becomes smaller as p becomes closer to either 0 or 1. When p nears 0 or 1, almost all the N events will result in the same outcome. As a result, there will be very little variability in the experiment when p is extreme. The largest variance, and greatest uncertainty about the outcome, occurs when $p = 1/2$. A special case of the binomial distribution for large values of N and small values of p is discussed in Chapter 10 on the Poisson distribution.

When we conduct a binomial experiment and observe the number of successes x, then we usually estimate p by x/N or the empirical fraction of observed successes. We must be careful to distinguish between the unobservable probability p and its estimated value. For this reason, we usually denote the estimate as $\hat{p}$, where the caret signifies an estimate of the unknown quantity. We read the expression $\hat{p}$ as "p hat."

The mean of $\hat{p}$ is equal to p so we say $\hat{p}$ is an *unbiased* estimator for p. The standard deviation of $\hat{p}$ is equal to $\sqrt{p(1 - p)/N}$. It is common practice to replace the ps in this expression by $\hat{p}$ itself, resulting in an estimated standard deviation. (We recall from Section 1.1 the standard deviation is the square root of the variance.)

Our uncertainty associated with the unknown parameter p can be expressed in terms of its estimator $\hat{p}$ and its estimated standard deviation

$$\sqrt{\frac{\hat{p}(1 - \hat{p})}{N}}.$$

We can also express our uncertainty about the unknown p parameter in terms of a *confidence interval*. A 95% confidence interval for the binomial p parameter is

$$\left(\hat{p} - 1.96\sqrt{\frac{\hat{p}(1 - \hat{p})}{N}}, \quad \hat{p} + 1.96\sqrt{\frac{\hat{p}(1 - \hat{p})}{N}} \right). \tag{2.4}$$

A confidence interval, in general, expresses our uncertainty about the true parameter value in terms of an interval combining the sampling error and the idea of repeating the basic experiment. In the present case, if we repeated the binomial experiment many times and N was always the same large number, then we would find the distribution of all of the estimated $\hat{p}$s would look approximately like the normal or bell curve. (More details on the normal distribution are given in Section 2.3.)

Just as 95% of the normal curve is contained between the mean minus 1.96 standard deviations and the mean plus 1.96 standard deviations, it follows the true value of the parameter p should be contained in this interval 95% of the time. This is a fairly long list of assumptions because we (1) have only one sample, not many, and (2) the value of N is not necessarily large in most cases. Nevertheless, the confidence interval for p given here is a well-accepted way to express our uncertainty about this parameter.

Let's work out a numerical example in **R**.

Output 2.1 Code to generate binomial confidence intervals.

```
> prop.test(x=16, n=28, correct = FALSE)

1-sample proportions test without continuity correction

data:   16 out of 28, null probability 0.5
X-squared = 0.57143, df = 1, p-value = 0.4497
alternative hypothesis: true p is not equal to 0.5
95 percent confidence interval:
 0.3907079 0.7349145
sample estimates:
        p
0.5714286


> prop.test(x=16, n=28)

1-sample proportions test with continuity correction

data:   16 out of 28, null probability 0.5
X-squared = 0.32143, df = 1, p-value = 0.5708
alternative hypothesis: true p is not equal to 0.5
95 percent confidence interval:
 0.3743185 0.7497305
sample estimates:
        p
0.5714286
```

Suppose we observe $X = 16$ successes out of $N = 28$ trials. In Output 2.1, we obtain a 95% confidence interval for the binomial p parameter. The 95% confidence interval using the normal approximation in (2.4) is (0.39, 0.73). Another binomial confidence interval uses the continuity corrected chi-squared and obtains the interval (0.37, 0.75). In either case, the single point estimate for p is $16/28 = 0.57$. The **R** codes in these two examples both use the prop.test function, with and without the correct= option.

The continuity-corrected chi-squared is described in Section 2.6. The prop.test function also performs a hypothesis test concerning the p parameter. Hypothesis tests are reviewed in Section 2.4.

The continuity correction was proposed because statistical workers sometimes felt uncomfortable using the normal approximation to the binomial distribution with small sample sizes. A simple correction would make a smaller error due to this approximation.

Is it possible to obtain a confidence interval with *no* approximations at all? The answer is *yes* and it relies on the computer power we have today which was not available at the time these earlier methods were used. Let us work out an example for the present data values.

We continue the example given in Output 2.1 with $X = 16$ successes out of $N = 28$ trials. We want to find the range of values of the p parameter so 95% of the probability covers the observed value of 16.

Specifically, let us search for the values of (p_1, p_2) solving the pair of equations

$$\Pr[\, X \geq 16 \ \text{for parameter value } p_1 \,] = 0.025$$

and

$$\Pr[\, X \leq 16 \ \text{for parameter value } p_2 \,] = 0.025.$$

Both of these equations ask us to find values of the p parameter giving probability 0.025 to each of the two tails of the distribution of the observed value $X = 16$.

A little trial and error gives us

```
> sum(dbinom(16:28, size = 28, prob = .3718))
[1] 0.0250042
> sum(dbinom(0:16, size = 28, prob = .7554))
[1] 0.02498158
```

so the required confidence interval is $(0.372, 0.755)$.

Notice how we found this confidence interval without appealing to any approximations, normal or otherwise. Such methods are referred to as *exact*. Exact methods do not offer a higher virtue, but rather lack any assumptions beyond those expressed by the underlying binomial distribution. The exact method used in this example is performed easily with a little trial and error but would represent a huge effort if this had to be performed by hand. Finally, notice how this last confidence interval is not very different from the two results obtained in Output 2.1.

The reader is encouraged to work out another example in Exercise 2.9. Other exact methods are described in Section 2.6.

2.2 Confidence Intervals and the Hubble Constant

Einstein's mathematics gave theoretical evidence the universe is expanding, but it wasn't until 1929 that Edwin Hubble[2] provided the empirical evidence for this. Even more remarkable was the claim the farther galaxies were from us, the faster they were moving away. The current estimate is objects 3.3 million light years farther away are moving 74 km/s faster. The exact rate, called the Hubble constant, is important to cosmologists and so much depends on it. Will the universe keep expanding following

---

[2] Edwin Hubble (1898–1953), American astronomer. The Hubble Space Telescope carried into orbit in 1990 was named after him.

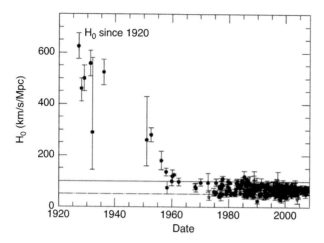

Figure 2.2 Estimates and confidence intervals for the Hubble constant over time. *Source:* John Huchra and the Harvard–Smithsonian Center for Astrophysics.

the Big Bang, or will it reach a maximum and then come back together again because of gravity? Cosmologists now say the Hubble quantity is not really constant, because gravity will slow the expansion but dark energy will speed it up over long periods of time.

Over time there have been different estimates as scientists use increasingly sophisticated methods. There were also a few estimates before Hubble's in 1929. The estimates of the Hubble constant, along with their corresponding confidence intervals, are plotted in Fig. 2.2. The earlier measurements had larger confidence intervals, and these did not always overlap one another. More recently, increasingly precise instruments have been used, and these provide smaller confidence intervals. The present estimates all fall in the range of 50 to 100. Figure 2.2 shows the history of the Hubble constant and demonstrates how a consensus is being reached.

Two statistical methods can be used to examine data such as given in this figure. Both methods are beyond the scope of this book but can be explained briefly here. The first of these methods is called *meta-analysis*. Meta-analysis seeks to combine different sources of information in order to obtain a single estimate. In the present example, different experimental methods were used to estimate the Hubble constant, and these are based on different sources of empirical data. Some of these are clearly less precise than others, but still have some value in obtaining the final estimate. We might give some measurements more weight than others in our combined estimate, for example.

A second useful method for data such as these is *Bayesian statistics*. A statistician employing Bayesian methods would express uncertainty about the Hubble constant in terms of a statistical distribution with a mean and a standard deviation. As more data is obtained, Bayesian methods show how to update this uncertainty, resulting in another statistical distribution. In this manner, the Bayesian approach demonstrates how we can improve on our knowledge of the Hubble constant by incorporating all of the prior knowledge and data accumulated to date.

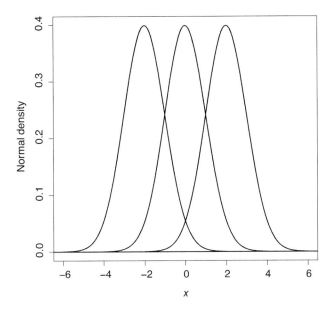

Figure 2.3 The normal distribution for means equal to −2, 0, and +2, all with a standard deviation of 1.

2.3   The Normal Distribution

The normal distribution is central to much of statistics. It is often referred to as the "bell curve" because of its shape. Its origins date back to de Moivre,[3] who used it in 1734 to approximate the binomial distribution. Today it is more often associated with the work of Gauss[4] about a century later. It is frequently referred to as the Gaussian distribution.

The normal distribution is characterized by its mean and standard deviation. When we change the mean, Fig. 2.3 shows the same shape is moved right and left. When we change the standard deviation, Fig. 2.4 shows it is either stretched or squeezed along the horizontal axis. The area under the normal curve is always equal to 1, so when the curve is squeezed, it must also rise in order to maintain the same area.

Notice, then, an important difference in the way the binomial and normal models are used. In the binomial distribution (Section 2.1), we can talk about the probability of a discrete event such as stopping at a traffic light six times. In contrast, the normal distribution is used for continuous outcomes.

Probabilities from the normal distribution must be described in terms of areas under the curve. Recall from Section 1.4, areas under a curve are usually found using calculus. The normal distribution is so popular there are many tables and software

---

[3] Abraham de Moivre (1667–1754). Mathematician and probabilist, born in France and later moved to London.
[4] Johann CF Gauss (1777–1855), German. One of most influential mathematicians. He also made many contributions to physics.

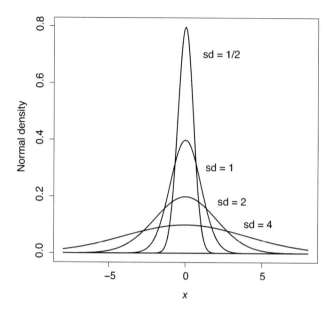

Figure 2.4 The normal distribution with mean 0 and different values of the standard deviation, as given.

packages available, and calculus is not necessary. In **R**, for example, we can use the pnorm function.

With so many possible means and standard deviations, how can any tables take into account all of the many normal distributions? The answer is we really need only have one normal curve, with a mean of 0 and a standard deviation of 1. This is referred to as the *standard normal* distribution. All normal distributions can be transformed into a standard normal by adding or subtracting (to get a mean of 0) and multiplying or dividing (to get a standard deviation of 1). More formally, if X is normal with mean μ and standard deviation σ, then

$$Z = \frac{x - \mu}{\sigma}$$

will behave as a standard normal.

Let us work out a few examples of using the function pnorm in **R**. The function pnorm(x) provides the area under the standard normal curve up to x in Fig. A.1 in the Appendix.

That is, this function provides the shaded area

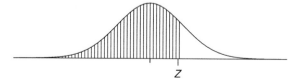

for all values of Z.

The Appendix provides more details of **R** functions for calculating areas in Fig. 1.3, but we will work out some simple examples here.

So, for example, we have

$$\Pr[\, Z \leq 0.62 \,] = 0.7323711,$$

found in **R** as follows,

```
> pnorm(.62)
[1] 0.7323711
```

To find $\Pr[\, Z \geq 0.92 \,]$, we note the shaded area in

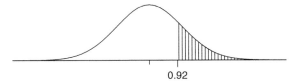

is 1 minus the shaded area in

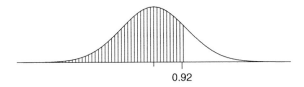

so

```
> 1 - pnorm(.92)
[1] 0.1787864
```

shows us

$$\Pr[\, Z \geq 0.92 \,] = 1 - \Pr[\, Z \leq 0.92 \,] = 0.1787864.$$

For a bigger example, we can find other areas such as

$$\Pr[\, -0.6 \leq Z \leq 1.4 \,]$$

using

```
> pnorm(1.4) - pnorm(-0.6)
[1] 0.6449902
```

namely, the area to the left of 1.4 less the area to the left of -0.6.

These rules can be combined to find other areas for normal distributions with different means and standard deviations. Exercise 2.7 asks the reader to find other normal probabilities for other settings.

We can find the inverse of the area as well. Specifically, the *quantile function* allows us to find the value of x for a given area. This function is called qnorm() in **R**. As an example, to find the quantile such that 85% area of the normal distribution lies below this point,

```
> qnorm(.85)
[1] 1.036433
```

giving the value 1.036.

2.4   Hypothesis Tests

One of the important roles of statistics is to provide convincing evidence of the validity (or falsity) of a certain claim about the nonobservable state of nature. Of course, statistical variability prevents us from saying a statement is 100% true, because we might just have observed an unusual sample of data. If we were only able to measure the heights of basketball players, for example, a reasonable conclusion would be all people are over six feet tall.

Even if we can safely assume our data is representative of the population, we still need to qualify our language with a certain measure of doubt about our conclusions. This is the framework of the hypothesis test.

You can think of a hypothesis test as a game we play with nature. We are presented with a choice of two different complementary statements about reality, referred to as hypotheses. Our job is to decide which is the true statement. Unlike a poker game, where we might have to risk a large sum of money in order to see if the other player is bluffing, in hypothesis testing we will never know if we made the correct decision. The objective is to pick the correct decision with high probability, even though we will never know with certainty which is correct. Figure 2.5 is a convenient way to illustrate all of the possible outcomes.

More specifically, a hypothesis test begins with a *null hypothesis* and a corresponding *alternative hypothesis*. The null hypothesis is typically a statement about the status quo, the way things are today. Examples might include stating a new way of doing things is no better or worse than the way we have been doing it all along. The new "Drug A" is the same as the standard treatment. "Brand X" detergent will get your clothes as clean as "Brand Y." These are examples of typical null hypotheses.

The alternative hypothesis is sometimes the opposite of the null hypothesis, so we might say Drug A is better or Brand X detergent makes clothes cleaner. In both

		Your decision:	
		Null hypothesis	Alternative hypothesis
Nature decides:	Null hypothesis	Correct decision	Type I error
	Alternative hypothesis	Type II error	Correct decision

Figure 2.5 A schematic of hypothesis tests. The significance level is the probability of incorrectly rejecting the null hypothesis. Power is the probability of correctly rejecting the null hypothesis.

examples we are expressing a *one-sided alternative hypothesis* – one in which a specified direction is of importance. Drug A is either better or not, so maybe we should rewrite the corresponding null hypothesis as "Drug A is at least as good as Drug B" and the alternative hypothesis as "Drug A is better."

There are also *two-sided alternative hypothesis tests* of interest in settings where we are interested in whether or not a change has occurred and we have no particular stake in the direction of the change. Suppose we are manufacturing a generic drug and want to show it is equivalent to the original. In this case, any change, regardless of direction, will show the new generic is different.

The alternative hypothesis is more often expressed in terms of a quantitative difference from the null. So, for example, valid alternative hypotheses might be Drug A will result in patients having 20% fewer colds this winter and Brand X will make your clothes 30% brighter as measured in terms of reflected light. The two-sided generic drug example might be willing to tolerate a difference of up to 10% response rate.

The reason for quantifying the difference between the two hypotheses is to specify the actual magnitude of a meaningful difference. If the difference is too small to be experienced, then it is probably not worth our while to convince others which of the two hypotheses is more likely to be valid.

The next step is to identify a statistical measure of the difference between these two hypotheses. After washing several piles of clothes, we measure the light reflectivity under two different detergents and then compare the two averages using the t-test, described in Section 2.5. Similarly, we might ask two groups of patients to take either Drug A or a placebo and then report back in the spring on the number of colds they experienced over the winter. We might look at the difference in the two rates.

How large should these differences be? Under the null hypothesis of no difference, the differences should be rather small. Of course, the size of the difference would depend on such factors as the sample sizes involved, the precision of our light meter, and the memories of our patients. Even after taking all of these factors into account, there will still be observed differences, and we will need to quantify the magnitude of these.

The magnitude of the difference is often expressed as the probability such a difference could have occurred by chance alone under the null hypothesis. This probability is called the *p-value*. The *p*-value is a measure of how unusual the observed outcome would be if all the conditions of the null hypothesis were valid. The *p*-value is also known as the *significance level* or *statistical significance*.

> Statistical significance is the probability such an outcome could have occurred by chance alone under the null hypothesis.

What often happens in practice is the author of an experiment will only report the *p*-value and leave it up to the reader to figure out what the null and alternative hypotheses are. Some journals publishing scientific studies are now asking authors to spell out these hypotheses. Similarly, every time we hear the expression "*p*-value," we should always be ready to ask about the null hypothesis if it is not immediately obvious from the context.

Let us return to the interpretation of a *p*-value. If an unusually small *p*-value is reported, it means something unusual has occurred under the null hypothesis. At this point we will usually conclude the null hypothesis is not valid and use the *p*-value as evidence for the alternative. More formally, we are said to *reject the null hypothesis* in favor of the alternative. Intuitively, if something very rare has just occurred, then we are moved to say something must be wrong in our thinking. In this case, a small *p*-value suggests perhaps the null hypothesis is not the correct explanation for the observed data.

Notice the *p*-value is not the probability the null hypothesis is true. This is a common misinterpretation of the *p*-value. The *p*-value is a measure of how tolerant we may be of unusual outcomes. This tolerance will vary depending on the circumstances. Another popular misconception is observed values of *p* smaller than 0.05 are the only times we would reject the null hypothesis.

Although 0.05 is certainly a popular value, observing an outcome occurring only 1 in 20 times need not cause us to reject an assumption held up to close scrutiny. Consider a situation where we are examining a newly developed, but largely unstudied, technology or drug which may show great promise in the future. We may not be able to devote a lot of resources to testing it on a large sample size. In this situation we might use a more generous criterion to reject the null hypothesis the new method is not any better than the current standard method. Failing to reject the null hypothesis in this setting may result in a potentially great idea being discarded too early in its development. If we use a *p*-value of 0.10, for example, then we are giving the new idea a generous benefit of the doubt.

At the other extreme, if we have a huge amount of data available to us, then we will need to have very strong evidence before we start making judgments and generalizations. Consider research based on the Surveillance Epidemiology and End Results (SEER) database. This program began in 1973 and is presently a complete census of all cases of cancer occurring in 18 states and metropolitan areas across the United States. With such a huge sample size, we are able to test even the most subtly different pair of hypotheses with a very high probability of choosing the correct one. Unfortunately, such close hypotheses may not be meaningful. Obtaining an extreme level of significance may not translate into a clinically recognizable advantage. An increase in lifespan measured in hours is not useful, regardless of how statistically significant the results may appear.

This leads us to the other problem of hypothesis testing seen in Fig. 2.5, namely failing to reject the null hypothesis when appropriate. We need the ability to detect a difference when one actually exists. Just as with the uncertainty measured by the *p*-value (the probability of incorrectly rejecting the null hypothesis) the *power* is the probability of correctly rejecting the null hypothesis when the alternative is true. Again, refer to Fig. 2.5 to clarify these two different errors.

> Power is the probability of correctly rejecting the null
> hypothesis when the alternative is true.

Power is more difficult to measure because it depends on the specific alternative hypothesis under consideration. Intuitively, if the null and alternative hypotheses are further apart in some sense, then less information is needed to tell the difference, and the power should be greater. In the abstract, it is easier to tell the difference between black and white than between two closely tinted shades of gray.

Let us take a more concrete example to illustrate this point. Suppose, in this example, we have a new method for predicting tomorrow's weather. The best methods available today are accurate 60% of the time. It will take us a very long time to prove the benefits of the new method if it is only accurate 62% of the time. This 2% improvement will be difficult to see unless we apply our new method for quite a long while. That is, the power, or the probability of detecting the improvement, will be very low in this problem unless we are willing to invest a lot of time and energy into studying it.

Of course, some may argue improving the accuracy from 60% to 62% is hardly worthwhile. Even if we had enough historical data and could claim an extreme statistical significance level (i.e., a very small p-value), there may be little to be gained if many people use the old forecasting method and would be reluctant to change. This is another example of clinical versus statistical significance: The amount of improvement is too small to be experienced despite claims of statistical significance.

We can increase the power in the forecasting example by considering an alternative hypothesis in which we claim the new forecast is accurate 80% of the time. There is a trade-off with this approach. Although the difference between the old method with 60% accuracy and the new method with 80% accuracy is a greater improvement, we are also making a much larger claim the new method must achieve. In words, we have greater power for testing hypotheses further apart, but at the same time, the method being tested must clear a much larger hurdle.

Let us end this section with a discussion of multiple comparisons. In the IMF/TB example described in Section 1.6, we pointed out a large number of diseases might have been compared across the IMF loan and nonloan nations. What effect might these multiple comparisons have on the final results presented?

Suppose every disease compared would be declared statistically significant at the 0.05 level. This means under the null hypothesis (there is no difference between the loan and nonloan nations), there is a 5% chance of rejecting the null hypothesis. If we did this for two different diseases, would there still be a 5% chance of rejecting at least one null hypothesis for either of these diseases?

The answer is no. Two actions have occurred, each with probability 0.05 of occurring. The chance at least one occurred will be greater than 5%. It is not clear exactly what the probability would be, but the chances of at least one being found statistically significant is going to be larger than 0.05.

As an extreme example, if 100 diseases were compared, then there we would expect a difference would be found in about five of these at the 0.05 significance level.

What is the appropriate significance level to cite in this case? The answer to this question is not easy, because it is not clear whether or not the different diseases occur independently or not. A large number of TB cases might be associated with a high rate of other lung diseases, for example.

One way to correct for the multiple comparisons is to divide the necessary significance level by the number of comparisons being made. This is called the *Bonferroni*[5] *correction* to the significance level. In words, if two disease comparisons are made, then we must attain a statistical significance of $0.05/2 = 0.025$ on either of these in order to claim an overall 0.05 significance level. The overall significance rate in this case is sometimes referred to as the *false discovery rate.*

In the examples discussed in this book, we do not need to be concerned with the Bonferroni correction to significance tests. The examples we examine are exploratory and used to illustrate the statistical methods involved. In serious scientific examination, however, we need to be aware of such false discovery biases and correct for them. As an important example, when a developer of a new drug seeks US Food and Drug Administration (FDA) approval and makes several claims for their product, they need to carefully document the overall statistical significance for each of these claims to show these are not overstated.

2.5   The Student t-Test

The Student t-test is the most commonly used method for statistically comparing the means of two different normal populations. The method assumes there are two populations, both with normally distributed attributes. Observations are independently sampled from each of these populations. We want to compare the means of the populations by looking at the differences of the two sample averages.

> The Student t-test is used to draw statistical inference on the difference of means of two normal populations.

If the sample averages are very different, then we can reasonably conclude the population means are different as well. The null hypothesis is the two populations have equal means, and the alternative hypothesis is the underlying means are different.

The difference in the sample averages needs to be standardized by an estimate of the standard error. We usually assume the standard deviations are the same in both of the underlying populations, but there are adjustments **R** can make if you think this may not the case.

The *Student t-distribution* is used to describe the behavior of the standardized difference of two sample means. The process of standardization requires the difference

---

[5] Carlo Emilio Bonferroni (1892–1960), Italian mathematician.

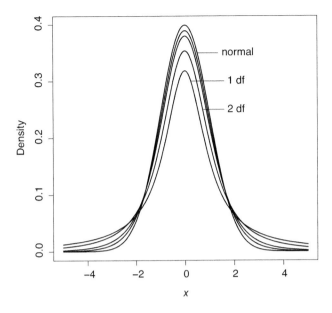

Figure 2.6 Student t-distributions with 1, 2, 5, and 10 df, and the normal distribution.

of the two averages to be divided by an estimate of its standard deviation. In a case where the population standard deviations are the same, Fig. 2.6 shows the distribution of the test statistic. These distributions are indexed by the degrees of freedom (df), which are 2 less than the number of observations in the two combined samples. As we can easily see, the larger the sample size, the more the Student t-distribution looks like a normal. The concept of degrees of freedom is discussed again in Section 2.7.

2.5.1   An Example in Practice

Let us work out an example. Consider this experiment on visual perception. The pair of boxes in Fig. 2.7 are a fusion set and initially appear to be sets of random dots. This is also called a random dot stereogram. On closer examination, these stereograms appear to be identical. If you hold the figure close to your nose and allow your eyes to slowly come in and out of focus, another pattern appears. This requires some time and patience. If you do this carefully and correctly, an embedded figure will appear to float above the background.

In a psychological experiment, two groups of volunteers were presented with fusion sets such as these. One group of subjects (NV) was given either a verbal message about the shape of the object or else no message at all. The other group (VV) was given this same verbal information and also shown a drawing of the embedded figure. The fusion times (in minutes) to resolve the images for each individual in these two groups are presented in Table 2.1.

The average fusion times of the groups of subjects were 8.56 min for the verbal-only group and 5.55 min for the verbal and visual subjects. The standard deviations

Table 2.1 Fusion times for two groups of subjects.

NV: Verbal message only									
47.2	22.0	20.4	19.7	17.4	14.7	13.4	13.0	12.3	12.2
10.3	9.7	9.7	9.5	9.1	8.9	8.9	8.4	8.1	7.9
7.8	6.9	6.3	6.1	5.6	4.7	4.7	4.3	4.2	3.9
3.4	3.1	3.1	2.7	2.4	2.3	2.3	2.1	2.1	2.0
1.9	1.7	1.7							

Average = 8.56   Standard deviation = 8.09

VV: Verbal and visual messages									
19.7	16.2	15.9	15.4	9.7	8.9	8.6	8.6	7.4	6.3
6.1	6.0	6.0	5.9	4.9	4.6	3.8	3.6	3.5	3.3
3.3	2.9	2.8	2.7	2.4	2.3	2.0	1.8	1.7	1.7
1.6	1.4	1.2	1.1	1.0					

Average = 5.55   Standard deviation = 4.80

Source: Frisby and Clatworthy (1975).
Online at https://dasl.datadescription.com/datafile/stereograms/.

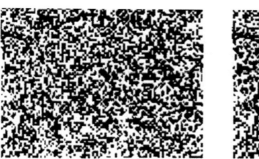 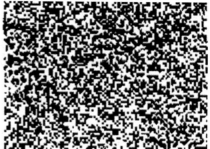

Figure 2.7 A random dot stereogram.

are 8 min and 4.1 min, respectively, in the two groups of subjects. These standard deviations are almost as large as the averages themselves, indicating there is considerable variability in the subjects' fusion times. Let us look at data values in Table 2.1. Most subjects resolved the fusion figure in a few minutes, but many struggled for more than 10 minutes. This suggests a right-skew to the data revealed in Figs. 2.8 and 2.9 in Section 2.5.2.

Let us recall some of the basic principles of statistics outlined in Section 1.1 before we go any further. Specifically, the observed data in Table 2.1 is a sample of empirical experiences based on a number of volunteers. These observations are sampled from an almost infinitely large population we will never be able to completely observe. The object of statistics is to use the observed, sampled data to make inferences about properties of the whole population.

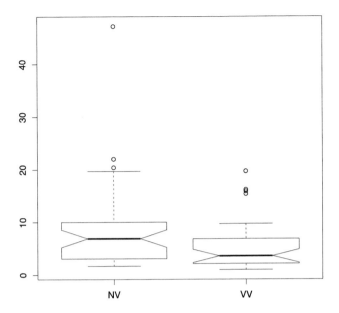

Figure 2.8 Boxplots for the fusion experiment.

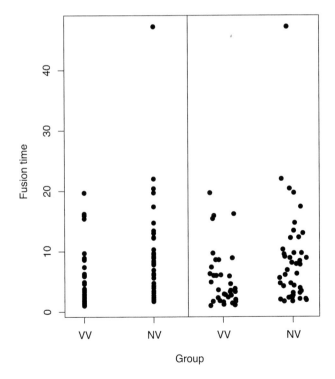

Figure 2.9 Fusion times by group and jittered group.

2.5.2   Read the Data and Perform Simple Checks

A small set of **R** instructions is given in Output 2.2 to read these data and produce some summary statistics. The data is read from a file called `visual_fusion.txt` from a file with headings. Specifically, the first few lines of `visual_fusion.txt` looks like this

```
Time Treatment
47.2    NV
22.0    NV
. . .
```

with useful column names. It is a useful habit to arrange your data in this fashion because the `header` = TRUE option carries the column names from this file into **R**.

Output 2.2 Program to read and produce simple statistics for a fusion experiment.

```
> fusion <- read.table(file = "visual_fusion.txt", header = TRUE)
> (last <- dim(fusion)[1])        # number of rows
[1] 78

> fusion[1:3, ]                   # first three rows
  Time Treatment
1 47.2        NV
2 22.0        NV
3 20.4        NV

> fusion[(last - 2): last , ]  # last three rows
   Time Treatment
76  1.2        VV
77  1.1        VV
78  1.0        VV

> (ind <- fusion[ ,2] == "NV") # T/F indicator for first group
 [1]   TRUE  TRUE  TRUE  TRUE  TRUE  TRUE  TRUE  TRUE  TRUE  TRUE  TRUE
[12]   TRUE  TRUE  TRUE  TRUE  TRUE  TRUE  TRUE  TRUE  TRUE  TRUE  TRUE
[23]   TRUE  TRUE  TRUE  TRUE  TRUE  TRUE  TRUE  TRUE  TRUE  TRUE  TRUE
[34]   TRUE  TRUE  TRUE  TRUE  TRUE  TRUE  TRUE  TRUE  TRUE  TRUE FALSE
[45] FALSE FALSE FALSE FALSE FALSE FALSE FALSE FALSE FALSE FALSE FALSE
[56] FALSE FALSE FALSE FALSE FALSE FALSE FALSE FALSE FALSE FALSE FALSE
[67] FALSE FALSE FALSE FALSE FALSE FALSE FALSE FALSE FALSE FALSE FALSE
[78] FALSE

> print(c( mean(fusion[ind, 1]), sd(fusion[ind, 1])))    # mean, sd for NV
[1] 8.560465 8.085411

> print(c( mean(fusion[!ind, 1]), sd(fusion[!ind, 1]))) # mean, sd for VV
[1] 5.551429 4.801738
```

The variable `fusion` contains the data in two columns, namely the fusion times and the name of the group, either NV or VV. The process of reading your data into **R** is a very common source of error. It is always a good idea to print out the first and last few observations to see if everything is being done correctly, as illustrated in Output 2.2.

After reading the data and convincing ourselves this was done correctly, we create the indicator variable `ind` with `TRUE` and `FALSE` values to distinguish the two different treatment groups. We print this out as well just to make sure it was created correctly.

Another good habit to get into is to document or explain the various steps of your code as you write it. Everything on a line following the `#` sign is treated as a comment.

Before we proceed with the statistical examination of any data, it is always useful to plot the data to see if there are any things we can quickly learn. A useful graphical display for these data is the *boxplot*. This figure was produced using the command

```
boxplot(Time ~ Treatment, data = fusion, notch = T)
```

in **R**.

The medians are depicted by horizontal lines inside the center of each box. The *median* is the value dividing the sample in half: half of the observed data are above this value and half are below. The notch in the center of the boxplot is a 95% confidence interval for the median. Statistical methods for comparing medians are given in Section 7.1.

The tops and bottoms of the boxes locate the upper and lower *quartiles* of these data. The upper quartile is the point where 25% of the data is above and 75% below, with a similar definition for the lower quartile. The box extends from the lower quartile to the upper quartile and contains the location of the central half of the observed data. The notch in the center of the box is a 95% confidence interval for the median value. The *whiskers* are lines extending 1.5 times the inner quartile range above and below the quartile boxes. Anything outside these whiskers are considered extreme observations and plotted individually.

The boxplot allows us to perform a quick comparison of the data in these two groups. The medians and quartiles all look very similar. The most notable feature is the extremes extending above the boxes. These correspond to individuals who took a very long time to fuse their stereograms. The most extreme times occur in the NV group with no visual information about the image they were seeking.

In Fig. 2.9 we give a scatter plot for the fusion times by group membership. The left half of this figure is the raw data. The group membership is binary valued, and this results in two vertical stripes.

A bit more information can be seen when the group membership is *jittered,* or perturbed by a small amount of random noise. This noise is just enough to break up the pattern of the groups so we can see some of the patterns in the data. This allows us more easily to count the number of individual observations and identify patterns. In the jittered plot we can see the no-visual-image group (NV) has a single large outlier. The visual-image subjects in the VV group have generally smaller fusion times, but it contains a group of four whose times are slightly removed from the others.

The jittered plot can be produced using the following **R** code.

```
plot(jitter(ind+0), fusion[, 1], ylab = "Fusion time", pch = 19,
          xaxt = "n", xlab = "Group", cex.lab = 1.25)
   axis(side = 1, labels = c("VV", "NV"), at = c(0, 1))
```

The "x" values are the binary-valued group indicator variable ind plus a little normal random noise. The true/false values can also be used as 1/0 values in arithmetic operations. We add 0 to ind to make sure **R** interprets these values as numeric rather than logical values. The function rnorm() generates independent, standard normal values.

A close examination of Fig. 2.9 reveals a single large outlier in the NV group. Without this observation there does not appear to be much difference between the two experimental groups.

2.5.3   Run and Interpret the t-Test

The end of Output 2.2 shows there was a three minute difference in mean fusion times. Does a difference of three minutes in the observed averages suggest there is a difference in the underlying population mean times? Could we have observed such a large difference in average fusion times if it did not matter whether subjects were given the additional visual information? Is the observed difference of three minutes between the two group averages a measure of the effect of the visual prompting, or could this difference be attributed to chance alone? On the basis of this sampled data, what can we say about the populations? These statistical questions make inference on the population means and can be examined by using the t.test function in **R**. The program is given in Output 2.3.

The t.test program

```
t.test(fusion[ind, 1], fusion[!ind, 1], var.equal = T)
```

lists the values in the two groups to be compared. These are specified as the first column of the fusion times by fusion[,1]. The membership of the NV group ind or not !ind specify the rows of the data to be compared in the t-test. There is also an indication of whether we should consider the variances in these groups to be equal. The output from the t.test is given in Output 2.3.

The output from t.test begins with a number of statistics for the fusion time values. These include the value of the t-statistic used to compare to the distribution in Fig. 2.6, the number of degrees of freedom, and the corresponding p-value. The Welch test adjusts for fractional degrees of freedom to account for unequal variances if you include this option. The t.test program also provides a 95% confidence interval for the difference between the two group means and, finally, the values of the group means. When you run a program such as this, it is useful to verify the mean values coincide with those obtained previously.

Output 2.3 Program to compute the t-test comparing averages in the fusion experiment.

```
# t test, with equal vars
> t.test(fusion[ind, 1], fusion[!ind, 1], var.equal = T)


Two Sample t-test

data:  fusion[ind, 1] and fusion[!ind, 1]
t = 1.9395, df = 76, p-value = 0.05615
alternative hypothesis: true difference in means is not equal to 0
95 percent confidence interval:
 -0.0809383  6.0990099
sample estimates:
mean of x mean of y
 8.560465  5.551429


# t test, unequal variances
> t.test(fusion[ind, 1], fusion[!ind, 1], var.equal = F)


Welch Two Sample t-test

data:  fusion[ind, 1] and fusion[!ind, 1]
t = 2.0384, df = 70.039, p-value = 0.04529
alternative hypothesis: true difference in means is not equal to 0
95 percent confidence interval:
 0.06493122 5.95314037
sample estimates:
mean of x mean of y
 8.560465  5.551429
```

Recall the description of confidence intervals from estimates of the p parameter in the binomial distribution, discussed in Section 2.1. Confidence intervals provide a range likely to include the underlying population mean if many additional experiments were to be conducted. More informally, a confidence interval in the present example is likely to contain the true underlying and unobservable difference of population means.

In the top half of Output 2.3, we see the statistics comparing the averages of the two groups of subjects in the fusion experiment assuming the variances are the same in the two populations. This method yields a p-value of 0.05615 providing a moderate amount of evidence the two population means are not equal.

Based on the discussion in Section 2.4, there is no way we will ever know this for certain. Instead, the p-value for this t-test is the probability of observing such a large difference in the sample averages if we assume:

- The two populations are sampled from underlying normal distributions;
- the two populations have the same means and variances; and
- the subject times are independent.

The alternative hypothesis is the two groups of subjects have different means. The p-value tells us the probability is 0.05615 of observing such a large difference, or larger, in the two sample averages when all these assumptions hold.

There are also variations of the t-test used when the variances are not equal and there are several ways of performing this test. The Welch–Satterthwaite method adjusts the degrees of freedom to account for unequal variances. This method gives a p-value of 0.04529, or just slightly smaller than the p-value obtained when we assumed the population variances are equal.

These p-values are fairly close and both provide about the same moderate amount of evidence the null hypothesis should be rejected. In conclusion, there is some evidence the populations have different means on the basis of the observed data. It appears visual information shortens the fusion time it takes people to resolve a random dot stereogram.

A p-value of 0.05 is not an automatic threshold for us to reject the null hypothesis, especially when these two methods yield p-values so close in value. A change in the basic assumptions gave rise to a relatively small change in the resultant p-value. This should not result in an abrupt change in our actions if a threshold is breached as a result of our change in assumptions.

Is there a statistical test of equality of variances? Yes. In fact, there are several. A commonly used example is the var.test, and its use appears in Output 2.4.

The var.test examines the ratio of two variances. The null hypothesis is: the ratio of variances is unity. The test in Output 2.4 provides a 95% confidence interval for this ratio. The test also provides a p-value of 0.0023, providing strong evidence the variances of the two groups are not equal. In the present example, Fig. 2.9 shows the differences in the variances may be due to a single outlier. This single outlier may also significantly contribute to the difference in the means.

Output 2.4 Test for equality of variances in the fusion time experiment.

```
> var.test(fusion[ind,1], fusion[!ind,1])   # test equality of variances

F test to compare two variances

data:  fusion[ind, 1] and fusion[!ind, 1]
F = 2.8354, num df = 42, denom df = 34, p-value = 0.002345
alternative hypothesis: true ratio of variances is not equal to 1
95 percent confidence interval:
 1.464690 5.367178
sample estimates:
ratio of variances
          2.835354
```

Are the fusion times normally distributed? One subject took a very long time to resolve the figure. This provides evidence the underlying distribution of fusion times in the general population may have a nonnormal distribution.

To summarize our examination of these data, there is moderate evidence of a difference in fusion times. There is one large outlier in the NV group providing considerable influence in this difference as well as the difference in the variances. If we rely only on the p-value from the t-test, then we conclude statistical significance. This is especially true if we tailor our test and choose to report only the result of the test for unequal variances. If we look at Fig. 2.9, however, it is possible this difference can be attributed to the influence of the single outlier in the NV group.

The larger question is whether we should rely entirely on computer-generated tests of hypotheses such as p-values and confidence intervals. Don't blindly cite the generated statistics without spending the time to convince yourself of the validity of the underlying assumptions. Look carefully at the data and consider how it was generated. This might tell us a different story. We saw this problem with the example presented in Section 1.6.

> Statistics is more than reported p-values.
> We still have to look at the data and think for ourselves.

Other approaches to comparing two groups of subjects to minimize the influence of a few outliers are considered again, in Chapter 7. One less than satisfying approach is to simply omit the outlier and start again. But then should we always delete data failing to conform to our expectations? Suppose we learned there were additional volunteers, not reported here, who were unable to identify the hidden figure and gave up looking. How should we examine their data?

Exercise 2.10.4 suggests we consider a transformation of the original data. Exercise 7.6 uses a different approach which reduces the effects of nonnormally distributed data and the influence of a few unusual observations. Other aspects of this experiment are discussed in Exercise 2.4.

To end this section, let us provide a historic footnote to the question: Who was "Student"? His real name was William Sealy Gosset (1876–1937). He worked as a quality engineer for the Guinness Brewery in Ireland in the early 1900s. His development of the t-test was considered a trade secret by his employer, and he was not allowed to publicize his work. In order to publish his result and at the same time hide his identity, Gosset chose to publish his t-test in 1908 under the pen name "Student." Eventually he was found out, but the pen name remains. To this day, the well-known t-test is attributed to Student, rather than to the true name of its discoverer.

2.6   The Chi-Squared Test and 2 × 2 Tables

One of the most common ways to describe the relationship between two different binary-valued attributes measured on each individual is to summarize these as

Table 2.2 Incidence of tumors in mice exposed to Avadex.

	Exposed	Control	Totals
Mice with tumors	4	5	9
No tumors	12	74	86
Totals	16	79	95

Source: Innes *et al.* (1969).

frequency counts in a 2 × 2 table. An example is given in Table 2.2. This table summarizes an experiment in which 95 mice were either exposed to a fungicide (Avadex) or kept in unexposed, control conditions. After a period of time, all mice were sacrificed and examined for tumors in their lungs. The aim is to describe any association between fungicide exposure and the presence of lung cancer.

This table displays the discrete numbers of exposed and unexposed mice, as well as those with and without lung tumors. The totals in the margins of this table also provide the numbers of exposed (16) and unexposed (79) mice, as well as the overall numbers of mice with tumors (9) and those without tumors (86). These are sometimes referred to as *marginal counts* because they ignore the effects of the other variable in the table.

Such 2 × 2 tables are popular in the scientific literature because they provide a concise summary of the data and allow us to examine the relationship between two attributes measured on each individual. In the present case, the attributes are exposure status (exposed or control) and tumor status (yes/no). Both of these are binary valued. If one of the attributes is continuous valued, then it is common practice to convert it into a binary-valued variable such as above or below the median value. In other words, even continuous-valued measures can be displayed in a 2 × 2 table.

The null hypothesis usually tested in a 2 × 2 table is that rows and columns are independent of each other. The expression of independence, by itself, is not intuitive until we translate it into the present context. In the case of the data in Table 2.2, the two binary-valued measures are exposure (columns) and tumors (rows). Saying columns and rows are independent is the same as saying the rate of tumor formation is the same, regardless of whether the mouse was exposed to the fungicide. It is equally valid to say tumor formation is independent of exposure status.

We then might think the alternative hypothesis is *dependence*, but this is a poor choice of words. Similarly, the data in Table 2.2 cannot be used to prove exposure causes cancer. Causality is difficult concept and cannot be demonstrated in such a simple data summary. Instead, the alternative hypothesis is: Exposure and tumor formation are associated or correlated. Demonstrating this association is the best a statistician can do. It remains to the scientific community how to interpret this association and whether or not it is meaningful.

One simple measure of association is the *cross-product ratio* or *odds ratio*, calculated as

$$\frac{4 \times 74}{5 \times 12} = 4.93$$

for the data in Table 2.2.

A value near 1 is indicative of independence. A value of the odds ratio greater than 1, as in this case, shows a positive association. That is, exposure to the fungicide is associated with almost five-fold higher rate of tumor formation.

There are many methods for assigning a p-value to these claims of association between the rows and columns of a 2 × 2 table. One of the oldest and most widely used is the *chi-squared test* (chi is pronounced $k\bar{i}$, rhyming with "sky").

Use the chi-squared test to examine frequencies in a 2 × 2 table.

We calculate the chi-squared test by first finding the expected values of the counts under the null hypothesis of independence. The expected counts are found from the formula

$$\text{expected count} = \frac{(\text{row sum}) \times (\text{column sum})}{(\text{sample size})}. \tag{2.5}$$

As an example, the number of exposed mice with tumors is 4, and the expected number is

$$\frac{9 \times 16}{95} = 1.5\overline{1}6$$

so more were observed than expected.

The chi-squared statistic calculates the sum

$$\chi^2 = \sum \frac{(\text{observed} - \text{expected})^2}{\text{expected}} \tag{2.6}$$

over the four counts in the 2 × 2 table.

The value of this statistic is 5.408, calculated by **R** in Output 2.5. Just as with the t-statistic, these are indexed by the degrees of freedom. A 2 × 2 table has 1 df.

The observed χ^2 value of 5.408 corresponds to a p-value of 0.020. This p-value provides a good rationale for rejecting the null hypothesis of independence of exposure and tumor growth, and concluding these two attributes are somehow related to each other beyond what might happen by chance alone.

The printed `Warning message` in Output 2.5 is not as dire as it first appears. The approximation of the chi-squared statistic (2.6) by the theoretical *chi-squared distribution* is based on the assumption that all the expected counts are large. (The expected counts were described in (2.5).) The approximation of the p-value improves with larger expected counts. There is no absolute rule where the approximation suddenly becomes valid. The "larger than 5 rule" was suggested by W. Cochran[6] in the 1950s and remains with us to this day. **R** prints this warning to alert you of a potential problem.

---

[6] William Gemmell Cochran (1909–1980), statistician in Britain and the United States.

Output 2.5 The chi-squared test for Avadex data.

```
> (avadex <- matrix(c(4, 12, 5, 74), 2,2))   # express data as 2x2  matrix
      [,1] [,2]
[1,]   4    5
[2,]   12   74

> chisq.test(avadex, correct = F)              # Pearson chi-squared

Pearson's Chi-squared test

data:  avadex
X-squared = 5.4083, df = 1, p-value = 0.02004

Warning message:
In chisq.test(avadex, correct = F) :
  Chi-squared approximation may be incorrect

> chisq.test(avadex, correct = T)              # Yate's correction

Pearson's Chi-squared test with Yates' continuity correction

data:  avadex
X-squared = 3.4503, df = 1, p-value = 0.06324

Warning message:
In chisq.test(avadex, correct = T) :
  Chi-squared approximation may be incorrect
```

One approach to this approximation problem is to use a *continuity-adjusted chi-squared*, also known as the *Yates corrected chi-squared*. The continuity-adjusted chi-squared uses the formula suggested by F. Yates[7] in 1934,

$$x^2 = \sum \frac{(|\text{ observed} - \text{expected} | -0.5)^2}{\text{expected}},$$

and then compares this value with the chi-squared distribution.

The continuity-adjusted chi-squared is given in Output 2.5. Its value is 3.4503 with 1 df and it has a *p*-value of 0.0632. This *p*-value is somewhat larger than the *p*-value obtained from the unadjusted chi-squared.

Another common approach avoiding any approximation to account for small sample sizes is the *exact test*. To understand how the exact test works, consider the empty shell in Table 2.3 obtained by deleting the data of the fungicide experiment. We keep the same marginal counts of exposed/control and tumor/healthy animals as before but omit the actual data on the inside of the table.

---

[7] Frank Yates (1902–1994), British statistician.

Table 2.3 The underlying margins of Table 2.2 are the basis for exact tests.

	Exposed	Control	Totals
Mice with tumors	x		9
No tumors			86
Totals	16	79	95

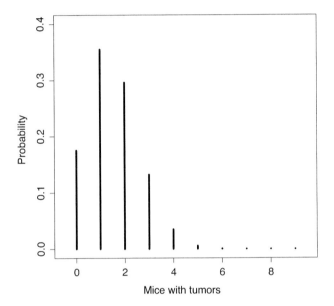

Figure 2.10 Exact distribution for the fungicide experiment under the null hypothesis.

Let us denote the number of exposed mice with tumors by the symbol x. In this table we see the value in this cell could assume any of the discrete values $0, 1, \ldots, 9$ consistent with the fixed marginal totals in this table. The observed value of x in the data is 4. More generally, if we assigned an arbitrary value to x in Table 2.3, then we could fill in all of the remaining cells of this 2 × 2 table. It does not matter which one of the four cells in the table we choose to assign a value; the other three entries would be similarly determined. The property one cell determines all others is discussed in Section 2.7, where the concept of degrees of freedom is explained.

The exact test for this table is based on listing all 10 of these possible outcomes and assigning a probability to each, without using an approximation or assuming very large sample sizes. These probabilities are plotted in Fig. 2.10. Exact tests are also referred to as Fisher[8] tests.

The observed value of $x = 4$ in this distribution has probability 0.0349. Importantly, we are not interested in the probability of this outcome but, rather, the

---

[8] Sir Ronald Aylmer Fisher (1890–1962), British geneticist, mathematician, and statistician.

probability of this or a more extreme outcome. That is, 4 *or more*, or perhaps, 4 *or fewer*. The concept of a *p*-value is the probability of the observed difference or larger, not the probability of the observed outcome. To repeat this concept, Exercise 2.5 points out an amusing conclusion reached when the method is misinterpreted.

The exact test will enumerate the probability of the observed outcome along with every other outcome more extreme. It is not clear what is meant by more extreme. There are two tails of the distribution in Fig. 2.10. A value of $x = 4$ or less has probability 0.9938, and a value of $x = 4$ or more has probability 0.0411. These two tail areas are obtained by specifying the tail area required in the fisher.test programs of Output 2.6. Notice these two probabilities do not add up to 1. Exercise 2.6 goes over this in detail.

We recognize 0.0411 to be the relevant tail area of this distribution and this is the exact significance level we report for these data. The **R** programs in Output 2.6 include exact confidence intervals for the odds ratios. These ratios are (0, 20.6) for the lower tail area and (1.07, +∞) for the upper tail. The confidence interval for the upper tail does not include the value of unity, corresponding to the null hypothesis of independence.

Output 2.6 The exact test for Avadex data.

```
> fisher.test(avadex, alternative = "greater")

Fisher's Exact Test for Count Data

data:   avadex
p-value = 0.04106
alternative hypothesis: true odds ratio is greater than 1
95 percent confidence interval:
 1.078304      Inf
sample estimates:
odds ratio
  4.814787


> fisher.test(avadex, alternative = "less")

Fisher's Exact Test for Count Data

data:   avadex
p-value = 0.9938
alternative hypothesis: true odds ratio is less than 1
95 percent confidence interval:
  0.00000 20.61462
sample estimates:
odds ratio
  4.814787
```

In conclusion, the exact p-value of 0.0411 falls in between the p-values obtained in Output 2.5 using the Pearson and Yates corrected chi-squared statistics. We can take this agreement as confirmation of the three different methods. In other words, there is moderate evidence of an association between the use of the fungicide Avadex and the development of lung tumors in mice.

All three methods (Pearson, Yates, and Fisher's exact) are commonly used in practice. The exact method is preferred with small sample sizes; use Pearson with large sample sizes; and Yates is a compromise.

The name "exact" appears to bestow a greater level of precision and transparency, but there is no real virtue in relying on these methods in every situation. In fact, it is generally recognized exact tests often suffer from reduced power and may fail to detect the alternative hypothesis when it is valid.

The chi-squared test and exact test will agree in large samples.
With small samples or when these tests are discrepant, use the exact test.

With large sample sizes, the exact and chi-squared tests will come to roughly the same conclusions, as in the fungicide example. The conclusions of these three tests will be in better agreement as the sample size increases. If there is a large discrepancy in a small sample, then we should rely on the exact test.

2.7 What Are Degrees of Freedom?

What exactly are degrees of freedom? We have seen this curious expression in two settings now: in the use of the t-test and when using the chi-squared test.

Let's look at two situations where these words come up. The expression

$$\sum_{i}^{N} (x_i - \overline{x})^2$$

(where $\overline{x}$ is the average of the x_is), is associated with $N - 1$ degrees of freedom.

Similarly, in a 2×2 table of counts, we always say the chi-squared statistic has one degree of freedom.

The general rule is as follows.

Degrees of freedom are the number of data points
to which you can assign any value.

Let's see how to apply this rule. When we look at the expression $\sum(x_i - \overline{x})^2$, there are N terms in the sum. Each term is a squared difference between an observation x_i and the average $\overline{x}$ of all the xs. Let us look at these individual differences and write them down. We have

$$d_1 = x_1 - \overline{x}$$
$$d_2 = x_2 - \overline{x}$$
$$\vdots$$
$$d_N = d_N - \overline{x}.$$

There are N differences d_i, but notice these must always sum to zero. Adding all the values on the right-hand side gives a sum of the xs minus N times their average. The d_i must sum to zero no matter the values of the xs.

So how many differences d_i can we freely choose to be any values we want and still have them add up to zero? The answer is all of them, except for one. The last one is determined by all of the others so they all sum to zero. Also notice it does not matter which d_i we call the "last." We can freely choose $N - 1$ values and the one remaining value is determined by all the others.

Now let us examine the use of degrees of freedom when discussing the chi-squared test. As an example, let us return to the data given in Table 2.2. The chi-squared statistic measures the association of rows and columns. In the present example, the association of interest is between developing lung cancer and exposure to the fungicide. The test is independent of the numbers of mice allocated to exposure or not and the numbers of mice eventually developing tumors or not. The significance level of the test should only reflect the "inside" counts of this table and not these marginal totals.

Let us rewrite this table giving all the margins, but without the values on the inside. This appeared earlier as Table 2.3. In this table we see there are four missing numbers, but also notice any one of these determines the other three. If we knew the value of x (the number of exposed mice with tumors), for example, we could fill the whole table using our knowledge of the marginal totals.

It doesn't matter which of the four cells inside the table we call x. That is, any one value determines all the others. There is one degree of freedom in this table.

If we look at Table 2.3, we also see the count labeled as x can only take on the values $0, 1, \ldots, 9$, so there are exactly 10 possible outcomes consistent with these marginal totals. The Fisher exact test exploits this property and constructs a hypothesis test of independence by enumerating all 10 of these outcomes. The probabilities of these 10 possible events are plotted in Fig. 2.10. These are described for this example in Section 2.6.

2.8   R, in a Nutshell

Among the most frustrating experiences since the invention of computers is the human interactions with them. We are expected to remember passwords, endure long menus of options just to get a simple answer, be deluged by spam, read error messages and help files having no bearing on reality, and be patient when everything we have been working on for the past week has just vanished into thin air. Perhaps worst of all is the immediate feedback we receive when our intentions are misunderstood. There is no sense the computer gave a moment's consideration to our request, however patiently asked.

Having said all this, let us try to introduce **R**. First, you need to have **R** installed on your computer. You should also have a kind, understanding, patient friend nearby who is willing to drop everything at a moment's notice and show you where you went astray.

A great feature of **R** is the availability of the many application-specific packages written by **R** users. There is also an extensive help file. If you don't know the name of the feature you are looking for, there are several online forums probably addressing the subject and including examples.

If you don't already have **R** installed on your computer, there is a free download for most operating systems. At the time of this writing, the comprehensive **R** archive network (CRAN) is the place to look for a mirror site near you.

Also useful is the *RStudio*. RStudio is a collection of windows allowing you easily to write **R** code, submit the code, retrieve output, look at graphs, and get help on topics. Again, there is a free RStudio download you can install.

Open the RStudio program and you will see a set of four windows similar to those in Fig. 2.11. This figure includes work being done on the example in Section 2.6. In Fig. 2.11 we see the programs to run the exact test of the fungicide data and the **R** code to produce Fig. 2.10. The lower left window displays the output of the exact test and the lower right includes the figure. Let us describe the RStudio shell and then get back to **R**.

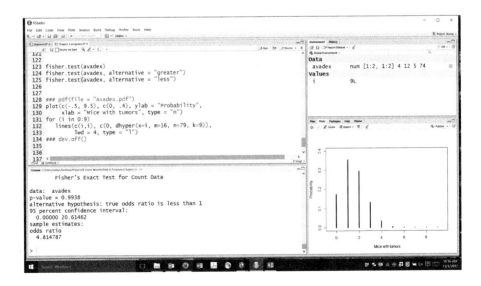

Figure 2.11 RStudio screenshot.

The upper left window of RStudio is a text editor. You can cut, paste, search, replace, and perform similar tasks with text here. There are tabs so you can have several documents open at one time and switch between them. Most of your code writing will take place in this upper left window. These tabs will open again after you turn your computer off and then return another day. To run **R** code, you highlight code in this window and press Ctrl-Enter.

The output of the submitted code appears in the lower left window. You can also type short commands in this window directly to work interactively in **R** but these commands are not saved for later.

The lower right window has tabs allowing you to switch between graphical displays and help files. The upper right window provides a list of all the data and variable names available to you.

The easiest way to learn a computer skill is to find a working program and then copy and modify it. The programs in this book are geared toward using this method of learning. After a while, you will want to consider additional options. When you reach this point, **R** offers an extensive Help File. Learn to use this valuable resource.

There are many useful reference books to teach you **R** as well as online tutorials. While we can't provide a comprehensive introduction here, we can work through a simple example. This example examines statistics on 100 low-birth-weight babies and will be examined in more detail in Chapter 3.

To begin, your data might look like the listing in Output 2.7. Every line in the data represents information on a single baby, and each of the seven columns represents a type of information, called a variable. The six variables in these data are (from left to right) head circumference; length at birth; gestational age; birth weight; mother's age; and an indication of pre-eclampsia. Pre-eclapmsia is a condition where the mother experiences high blood pressure and other disorders, which could lead to many complications including stroke.

Output 2.7 Contents of the low-birth-weight data file. Columns (left to right) are head circumference; length; gestational age; birth weight; mother's age; and an indicator for pre-eclampsia.

head	length	gage	wt	momage	pre.ecl
27	41	29	1360	37	0
29	40	31	1490	34	0
30	38	33	1490	32	0
. . . .					
28	35	32	880	35	1
28	41	33	1320	36	1
26	38	28	1080	36	0

Source: Pagano and Gauvreau (2000).

A typical **R** program reads the data including the column headings supplied in the data file. Be careful when reading data into **R**. This step is the greatest source of error. It pays to go over the coding carefully. Print out every step of the way to verify your work. Continue to print out every step until you are convinced your program is reading the data file correctly. Are the numbers in the correct columns? Is the last line of the file the same as the last line of the **R** data set?

> Be careful reading data into **R**. This is a common source of error.
> Print the results of every step to verify it was done correctly.

Everything after a # sign is a comment and ignored by **R**. Get in the habit of commenting on your programs so you will remember what you were doing long afterwards when you may have forgotten what your intentions were.

Let us look at the **R** statement in this script.

```
(leng <- dim(birthwt)[1])              # number of rows
```

The dim function returns the two dimensions of the data matrix birthwt. The first of these numbers is the length or number of rows. The subscript [1] refers to the first of these and the combination of characters <- assigns these to a variable we call leng. The whole statement is in parenthesis, so **R** will also print out this value.

A name on a line by itself (such as leng or birthwt) will print out its value. Typing birthwt[, 3:5] prints the data on the third, fourth, and fifth column variables (gestational age, weight, and mother's age).

The colon (:) produces a sequence of numbers. In this case 3:5 creates the list of values 3, 4, and 5. It is much less cryptic to refer to variables by name, as in birthwt$gage. Similarly, birthwt[3,] will print the third row of data.

The hist command produces a histogram. The xlab = code in Output 2.8 includes options to produce useful labels. The resulting histogram appears in Fig. 2.12.

The plot statement has many uses in **R**. The example reproduced in Fig. 2.13 is a *matrix scatter plot*. Every variable is plotted against every other variable, both on the *x*-axis and then on the *y*-axis.

Output 2.8 A short **R** program to read and examine the low-birth-weight data.

```
birthwt <- read.table(file = "birthwt.txt", header = TRUE)
(leng <- dim(birthwt)[1])              # number of rows
birthwt[1:3, ]                         # print first three rows
birthwt[(leng - 2) : leng, ]           # print last three rows
colMeans(birthwt)                      # means for each variable
hist(birthwt$wt, main = "Histogram of weights",
    xlab = "Weight in grams")
plot(birthwt, gap = 0, xaxt = "n", yaxt = "n") # maxtrix plot
```

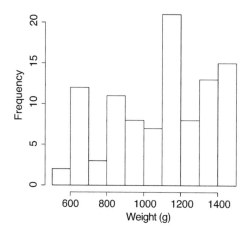

Figure 2.12 Histogram of baby weights.

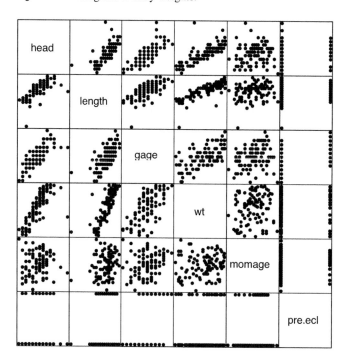

Figure 2.13 Matrix scatter plot for low-birth-weight babies.

2.9   Survey of the Remainder of the Book

Having reviewed the mathematical and statistical prerequisites, let us step back a moment and see what we are going to do with them and where we are going.

We begin with a data set measuring attributes on several individuals. The low-birth-weight infant data of Section 2.8 is a good example. The attributes or columns of these data are referred to as *variables*. Often one of these variables is of greatest importance to us, and we sometimes refer to it as the *outcome variable*. (Other books may refer to this as the *response variable* or *dependent variable*.)

The outcome variable is more important than any other data measured on each individual. We often refer to this variable by the symbol y because it is frequently plotted on the vertical axis. The object of this book is to show how we might explain the different values of the outcome variable y in terms of other information. Other variables measured on every individual are usually denoted by x and are sometimes called *independent variables* to distinguish them from the outcome y. We sometimes call y the *dependent variable* because its value will be explained using x. In the Chapter 3, we show how to explain the infant weight values y based on the length x of the infants. The concept of dependent variable is entirely a construct of our mathematical modeling framework and does not mean to imply a cause-and-effect relationship.

We begin with a detailed discussion of the situation where the response variable follows a normal distribution, in part because this is the most commonly encountered situation. Much research has gone into this setting and many diagnostics and graphical displays are available to facilitate the corresponding statistical analysis. Once we understand how to model the outcome as a normally distributed quantity, we can generalize to other settings where the outcome y might be binary valued, for example, or represent discrete counts.

Let us look back at the chi-squared test and t-test as examples. For the t-test, the outcome y has a continuous, normal distribution, and the explanatory or group membership variable x is binary valued.

In the chi-squared test in a 2×2 table, we might think of the row category explaining the column category or vice versa, and the dependent outcome variable (developing lung cancer or not) is binary valued. The explanatory variable (exposure or not to the pesticide) is binary valued in both of the chi-squared and t-test examples.

In the examples of all subsequent chapters, the explanatory variable can also be continuous. We demonstrate in those chapters how to combine the effects of multiple explanatory variables. For instance, the January temperatures in various cities (outcome) can be explained in terms of the latitude, as well as the altitude above sea level. We will need to combine the effects of latitude and altitude in explaining differences in temperature. One effect may be more important than the other, and we will need to assess the relative effects of other explanatory measures.

2.10   Exercises

2.1   I pass a certain intersection very often and have learned I will have to stop for the traffic light 65% of the time. If I pass through this intersection 12 times, use **R** to find the probability I will have to stop for the traffic light more than half the time.

2.2 There are eight preschool children in a day-care center. Suppose the probability is 1/4 one has a cold on given day.

a. Use the binomial distribution to estimate how many children you expect will have a cold on a given day. What is the standard deviation of this number?

b. What is the probability all eight children have a cold today? What is the probability three or more have a cold today?

c. Is this an appropriate use of the binomial distribution? Why or why not?

2.3 a. In a test of a hypothesis, does the power increase or decrease when the difference between the null and alternative hypotheses increases? Why?

b. Similarly, what kinds of alternative hypotheses have the greatest power? Should we consider these? Why?

c. What kinds of hypotheses can we test when the sample sizes increases? If the null hypothesis and the significance level remain the same, what kinds of alternative hypotheses can we test using the same level of power?

2.4 a. What is the population in the fusion experiment described in Section 2.5? Is it possible to consider examining every subject in the population?

b. Each subject was given either verbal-only or verbal and visual information. Should we be interested in what their outcomes might have been if they were randomized to the other group? If each subject was tested twice, once with verbal-only and once with verbal and visual information on different images, would it matter which condition was given first? What additional biases would this type of experiment introduce? In a *crossover experiment*, all subjects would experience both of the two different types of settings, but in a random order. That is, some would experience verbal only first and then the verbal and visual information whereas the others would receive these in the reverse order.

c. What evidence can you provide to suggest there were additional subjects who gave up and their data was not recorded? How would you take such information into account?

2.5 a. In the middle of a poker game, one of the players declares he holds a "kangaroo flush." His cards are 3◇, 6♡, 7♣, 9◇, and J♠. Of course there is nothing remarkable about this hand, but the player claims the probability of holding these exact five cards is extremely small. What is the probability of being dealt a kangaroo flush? On the basis of this extremely small probability, the player claims his cards must beat every other possible poker hand. What do you say about this argument?

b. Explain why the exact significance level of Table 2.2 is not the probability of observing this table. Instead, the significance level is the probability of observing this table or any other more extreme table.

c. List all the tables more extreme than the observed table. Show the odds ratios of these tables are larger than those of the observed table.

d. Following a lottery, somebody notices a pattern among the winning
    numbers such as: the four smallest numbers are all even. Can we use this
    type of observation to show the lottery is unfair? What is the null hypothesis
    in this case? More importantly, what is the alternative hypothesis? What is
    the probability somebody will say, "What is the probability of that?"

2.6   Why do the two tail probabilities add up to more than 1 in the exact test given in
Output 2.6? How do you interpret the sum of these two tail areas?

2.7   Use **R** to find the following probabilities for the normal distribution.

a. Find $\Pr[-2.18 < Z < 0.38]$ for a standard normal Z.

b. Find $\Pr[1.16 < Y < 2.72]$ for a normal Y with mean 1.35 and a standard
    deviation of 2.2.
    Hint: $(Y - 1.35)/2.2$ will behave as a standard normal, so we have

$$\Pr[1.16 < Y < 2.72] = \Pr\left[\frac{1.16 - 1.35}{2.2} < \frac{Y - 1.35}{2.2} < \frac{2.72 - 1.35}{2.2}\right]$$
$$= \Pr[-0.09 < Z < 0.62],$$

where Z behaves as a standard normal. We can also use options in the **R** function
pnorm() allowing for specification of different means and standard deviations.

2.8   In a clinical trial of chronic granulomatous disease (CGD, a hereditary immune
disorder), 128 patients were randomized to either a placebo or gamma interferon and
then followed for one year. Among the 63 interferon-treated patients, 14 experienced
at least one infection for a total of 20 observed infections. In the placebo group, 30
patients experienced at least one infection and 56 total infections were recorded.

a. Express the numbers of treated or placebo and infection-free or not as
    frequencies in a 2×2 table. Use the chi-squared test to see if gamma interferon
    was effective.

b. Would this be an appropriate way to compare the number of infections in the
    placebo and treated group?

c. Could we use the binomial distribution to compare the total number of
    infections? Here is how we might proceed: In total, $20 + 56 = N$ infections were
    recorded. Of the 20 infections in the treated group, these occurred in $\hat{p} = 63/128$
    fraction of the sample. How can we use the binomial model to obtain a p-value
    for these data? Comment on the validity of this approach.

2.9   Consider a binomial experiment resulting in 12 successes in 18 trials.

a. Estimate the value of the p parameter by maximizing (2.1) for $X = 12$ and
    $N = 18$. Use trial and error with the dbinom function in **R** to show the maximum
    occurs at $\hat{p} = 12/18 = 0.667$. This gives rise to expressing $\hat{p}$ as a *maximum
    likelihood estimator* because it maximizes the probability of the observed value.

b. Find an exact confidence interval for p with these data. Compare your results to
    those obtained using the prop.test function.

2.10   What is the hidden geometric shape in Fig. 2.7?

2.11   For every calendar day of the year and for many US cities, the National Weather Service website lists the highest and lowest recorded temperatures. When we look back in history and compare the years of these records, should the colder record occur earlier as often as the warmer record? If we compare every day of the year, is this a reasonable application of the binomial distribution with $N = 365$ and $p = 0.5$?

Specifically, in Washington DC, for 365 days of the year, there were 291 days in which the warmer record occurs more recently than the colder recorded temperature. What does the binomial distribution suggest for this observation? See Exercise 9.4.4 for more details on these data.

2.10.1   Maintaining Balance

It is difficult to maintain your balance when you are concentrating on something else. In an experiment involving aging, nine elderly volunteers (six men, three women) and eight young male volunteers tried to keep their balance while reacting to a randomly timed noise. They stood, barefoot, on a specially designed platform measuring their motion. Each time they heard the noise, they were supposed to press a hand-held button, all the while trying not to move. The data is given in Table 2.4.

Table 2.4 Measures of motion in a balance experiment.

	Motion		
Subject number	Forward and backward	Side to side	Age group
1	19	14	elderly
2	30	41	elderly
3	20	18	elderly
4	19	11	elderly
5	29	16	elderly
6	25	24	elderly
7	21	18	elderly
8	24	21	elderly
9	50	37	elderly
1	25	17	young
2	21	10	young
3	17	16	young
4	15	22	young
5	14	12	young
6	14	14	young
7	22	12	young
8	17	18	young

Source: Teasdale, Bard, LaRue, and Fleury (1993).

Table 2.5 Reading scores for third-grade children.

Additional directed activities									
24	43	58	71	43	49	61	44	67	49
53	56	59	52	62	54	57	33	46	43
57									

No additional activities									
42	43	55	26	62	37	33	41	19	54
20	85	46	10	17	60	53	42	37	42
55	28	48							

Source: http://lib.stat.cmu.edu/DASL/Stories/DRPScores.html.

Use a t-test to compare forward and backward motion distances in the elderly and young volunteers. Does age appear to make a difference in the responses? Use a t-test to compare these groups. Is there evidence the observed values are not normally distributed? Are there unusual observed values influencing the t-test? Should these be omitted, or should they be included in your examination of the data? Can you make an argument for both of these actions?

Repeat your examination using the side-to-side distances. Is your conclusion any different from the forward and backward motion?

How might we combine these separate measures of motion into a single number? Try it. You will need to define a new variable in your program. Print it out to make sure it is correct. Is your new measure useful in comparing the two groups of volunteers?

2.10.2 Reading Scores

Two groups of children participated in an experiment to see if their reading scores could be improved. One class of 21 children was presented with eight weeks of directed reading activities, and another control class did not receive this additional training. The scores from a standardized reading test are given in Table 2.5.

Did the additional directed reading activities improve the reading scores? Use a t-test and boxplot to support your conclusions. Do the test scores appear to be normally distributed within each of the two groups of children? Are the variances comparable? Is there any other information you would find useful in your analysis of these data?

2.10.3 A Helium-Filled Football

If we filled a football with helium, would a kicker be able to punt it farther? In an attempt to answer this important sports-related question, two identical footballs were presented to an amateur player who alternately kicked each as far as he could. He was unaware one football was filled with helium, the other with regular air from a pump. The kicking took place outdoors, on a windless day. The trial number and distances

Table 2.6 Distances two different footballs were kicked.

Trial	Air	Helium	Trial	Air	Helium	Trial	Air	Helium
1	25	25	2	23	16	3	18	25
4	16	14	5	35	23	6	15	29
7	26	25	8	24	26	9	24	22
10	28	26	11	25	12	12	19	28
13	27	28	14	25	31	15	34	22
16	26	29	17	20	23	18	22	26
19	33	35	20	29	24	21	31	31
22	27	34	23	22	39	24	29	32
25	28	14	26	29	28	27	22	30
28	31	27	29	25	33	30	20	11
31	27	26	32	26	32	33	28	30
34	32	29	35	28	30	36	25	29
37	31	29	38	28	30	39	28	26

Several sources, including: www.openintro.org/data/tab-delimited/helium.txt.

(in yards) kicked are given in Table 2.6. An internet search will reveal several videos of similar experiments, several involving professional players, some in front of a stadium full of viewers.

Why did the trials alternate between the two footballs? What biases would this remove from the experiment? The kicker did not know what the experiment was about. What biases would it introduce if he was told what was going on? A test subject who is unaware of the treatment is called *blind*.

Those evaluating the subject might provide unintentional or subtle messages about the experiment. An experiment in which those doing the evaluation are also blinded is called *double blind*. What biases might be avoided if those measuring the distance of the football kicks were also blinded as to the purpose of the experiment?

Plot the distances kicked by the trial number. Is there evidence the kicker improved as the experiment continued? Can you explain why this might be the case?

Look at a boxplot of the kicking distances for each of the two footballs. Is there evidence of extremely long or short kicks? Some might argue kicks of less than 15 or 20 yards are flubbed and should be neglected. Or maybe not.

What does the t-test tell us? Is there evidence of a difference between the two footballs? What other information would you find helpful in deciding if a helium-filled football provides an advantage in terms of kicking distance? Should a professional player be used, for example?

2.10.4   Reexamine the Fusion Times

Do the fusion times in Fig. 2.9 look normally distributed? What are the underlying assumptions we need to make in order for the t-test to yield valid inference?

Transform the fusion times using the `log` function in **R** and plot the fusion times. Do the log times appear more normally distributed? Repeat the t-test for the log-fusion times. Are your conclusions any different from those of Section 2.5.3?

Transformations of data are discussed again in Section 6.4. We will discuss non-parametric methods which allow us to analyze data without having to assume an underlying normal distribution in Chapter 7.

3   Introduction to Linear Regression

In this book we develop mathematical models for explaining the variability of measurements made on an outcome of interest. The aim is to try to explain the different values of this outcome in response to other information available to us. Random variation in the values of the response makes this difficult, and at best we will only be able to make a statement about the typical or average value of the response under a given set of circumstances. Let us make this clear with an example in which we try to explain the different birth weights of a group of 100 low-birth-weight babies using only information about their length.

3.1   Low-Birth-Weight Infants

Low-birth-weight infants may suffer from a myriad of health problems. Low birth weight is defined as any value lower than 1500 g. Figure 3.1 plots the length and birth weight of 100 low-birth-weight infants born in one of two Boston-area hospitals. The line through the figure provides an estimate of the weight for any given length. In Section 3.3 we describe the **R** code to draw this figure.

Figure 3.1 illustrates a general relationship between birth weight and length. For most babies, larger birth weight is associated with greater length. Despite a small number of notable exceptions apparent in this plot, we can see most of the infants follow a general pattern. The large "cloud" of observations along the right half of this figure defines the general pattern of the data. The values of length were rounded to the nearest centimeter, and this explains the vertical "stripes" appearing in Fig. 3.1.

The aim of this chapter and Chapter 4 is to fit the straight line to data and assess its adequacy in explaining the response. Of course a straight line is not going to explain the differences in all of the birth-weight values, but for a given value of length, we can make a statement about the average birth weight we should expect at that length.

Similarly, we are not making a prediction about the birth weight beyond suggesting where the average might be. *Prediction* is not a good word to use with this activity because we can only hope for an estimate of the typical observation under identical conditions.

We are also not trying to prove a cause-and-effect relationship. It would be foolish to try to prove greater length causes greater birth weight, or vice versa. Statistics alone cannot prove cause-and-effect relationships. In the present example, both length and

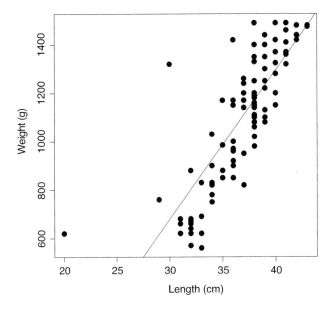

Figure 3.1 Birth weight and length of 100 low-birth-weight infants along with the fitted least-squares regression line.

birth weight are the result of other factors, and the cause-and-effect relationship is beyond the scope of this book. On the other hand, an infant's length can be estimated using readily available imaging technologies before birth, so it is a reasonable exercise to provide a good estimate of the ultimate birth weight.

The following section describes how the fitted line in this figure is determined.

3.2   The Least-Squares Regression Line

A line is determined by its slope and intercept. In this section we show how these two parameters are estimated from the data. Along the way, we also need to explain how the best-fitting line is going to be defined. All of the mathematical formulas and numerical calculations will be done in **R**. Even so, it is important for the user of these methods to understand the steps involved in fitting these mathematical models.

Let's introduce some notation. Our data consists of ordered pairs of coordinates:

$$(x_1, y_1), (x_2, y_2), \ldots, (x_n, y_n).$$

In terms of the low-birth-weight infants, the xs are the lengths and the ys are the corresponding birth weights. The aim of this section is to explain how to obtain a regression line model

$$y = \alpha + \beta x$$

for the data.

This equation is a mathematical model for the data. A quick look at Fig. 3.1 reminds us there is no reason for this line to pass through any of the data points. A model is a simplified version of reality. The line provides an intuitive summary of the relationship of weight and length for typical infants but is not indicative of any one of them.

A more accurate description of what is going on is to write a separate equation for each (x_i, y_i) pair. There is only one underlying line for the whole data set so there is only one intercept α and one slope β. We also need to consider that most data points do not lie exactly on this line. Some observations will be above the line and others will be below.

As a compromise, let us write

$$y_i = \alpha + \beta x_i + r_i,$$

where r_i is the difference between the observed value y_i and where it is expected to be if it appeared exactly on the line.

We call these r_i the *residuals* because they represent what is left over after fitting the line. In other words, there is one line with slope β and intercept α. At any given length x_i of the ith infant, the observed weight y_i will be close the estimated value on the line $\alpha + \beta x_i$. The residual is the difference between the observed value and where it would be expected if it appeared exactly on the line. The choice of best-fitting line is determined by these residuals. In Section 4.4 we will also see the residuals are useful in identifying any inadequacies of the model.

To determine the most appropriate line, we need to estimate both the intercept α and the slope β for this line. First, let's define a criterion by which we are to obtain these estimates. The process of estimation is motivated by the depiction of the data given in Fig. 3.2. In this figure we imagine the regression line passing near three data points, depicted by solid circles. The regression line is shown as a dotted line. This is an extreme close-up view of a very small part of the full data. There are many other data points, but these are outside the range of this figure.

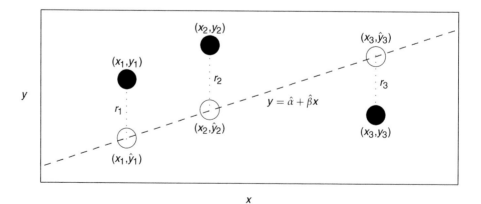

Figure 3.2 A close-up view of a small portion of the data and the regression model. Solid circles are the observed data. Open circles are their estimated values. The lengths of the vertical lines indicate residuals. The dashed line is the regression line.

For each of the three observations in Fig. 3.2, we can see where these observations would be if the line represented a perfect fit to the data. These perfectly fitted, or *estimated*, data points appear as open circles along the dashed line.

Note the residuals are expressed as deviations from the y values only. The estimated value is not identified as the closest point to the observed data on the regression line. The implications of this convention are the x values are assumed to be known to a high degree of precision and all statistical variability takes place along the vertical y axis. In the case of the low-birth-weight infants, for example, we assume the length is known with some degree of precision on the basis of a CT scan, and the infant's weight is the only variable we choose to explain.

> In linear regression we are estimating the mean
> of **y** for a known value of **x**.

The coordinate pairs of the estimated observation on the regression line are denoted by $(x_i, \hat{y}_i)$, where the carets ($\hat{\ }$) on the $\hat{y}$s are indicative of an estimated value. (We pronounce $\hat{y}$ as "y hat.") Similarly, the estimated intercept and slope are denoted by $\hat{\alpha}$ and $\hat{\beta}$, respectively.

Equally important in Fig. 3.2 are the *residuals* or differences between the observed and estimated values. Mathematically, we define

> residual = observed − expected

or how far the observed data is from where we would expect it to be in a perfectly fitting model.

The lengths of the three residuals are indicated by dotted lines in Fig. 3.2. Values of r_1 and r_2 are positive numbers because the observed data is larger than what the model expects; r_3 is negative.

In this and all subsequent chapters we see residuals play an important role in determining the adequacy of the models we build for data and help in identifying unusual observations in the data. Briefly, the residuals represent the shortcomings of a mathematical model in its representation of the observed data.

Let us look more closely at the residuals for our straight-line model. If we knew the values of the slope α and intercept β of the regression line, then the perfectly fitted observation corresponding to the observed pair (x_i, y_i) would be

$$\hat{y}_i = \alpha + \beta x_i$$

and the residual r_i is exactly zero because of the perfect fit.

That is, $\hat{y}_i$ is the value of y on the line at the value x_i. The values of $\hat{y}_i$ appear as the open circles in Fig. 3.2. We can write our definition of the ith residual as the observed y_i minus its expected value

$$r_i = y_i - \hat{y}_i$$

or as

$$r_i = y_i - (\alpha + \beta x_i). \tag{3.1}$$

This last representation of the residual will allow us to estimate the parameters α and β of the regression line. Ideally we would like all our residuals to be small in some sense. The principle of least squares provides the appropriate guidance on how to achieve this.

> Estimation using least squares minimizes
> the sum of squared residuals.

Using the guidance of least squares, the aim is to estimate α and β by minimizing

$$\sum_i (\text{residual}_i)^2.$$

Of course, we can't see α and β in this last expression, but if we look back at (3.1) we can write this as

$$\sum_i (y_i - \alpha - \beta x_i)^2. \tag{3.2}$$

The objective, then, is to find the values of α and β to minimize this quantity. We should immediately recognize this minimization as a problem from calculus. An overview of the principles of calculus appears in Section 1.4. We do not actually go through the details, but the reader should recognize the steps needed to be taken to solve the problem.

Specifically, we need to differentiate (3.2) with respect to α and set this equation to zero. We also need to differentiate (3.2) with respect to β and set this second equation equal to zero. These steps result in two equations in two unknowns: α and β.

These two equations are

$$\sum_i \text{residual}_i = 0 \tag{3.3}$$

and

$$\sum_i x_i \, \text{residual}_i = 0. \tag{3.4}$$

As written, again, we can't see the α and β, but they are there. Exercise 3.1 asks you to rewrite these two equations to make this clear.

There is no reason for us to solve these two equations: **R** does this for us. The computing is covered in Section 3.3, but it is important to see what **R** is actually doing in order to obtain the estimates $\hat{\alpha}$ and $\hat{\beta}$. Before that, let us describe the implications of these two equations.

Equation (3.3) asserts the residuals sum to zero or, more importantly, have an average value of exactly zero. Intuitively, this is a nice property. If the residuals represent the differences between the observed data and their expected values along the regression line, then we would want the line to represent the average values and not be either too high, on average, or too low. Equation (3.3) assures us the regression line is centered about the data. If $\bar{x}$ and $\bar{y}$ are the averages of the xs and ys, respectively, then the point of averages $(\bar{x}, \bar{y})$ is a point on the regression line.

The second equation (3.4) states the residuals are uncorrelated with the explanatory x values. We discuss correlation later in Section 4.1, but for the moment, the implication is the regression line contains all of the linear information that can be extracted from the explanatory variable. The least-squares regression line obtains all of the linear information available in the x values, and there is nothing left but the residual noise. A plot of the explanatory values (or fitted values) against the residuals of our model should show only random white noise with no apparent pattern or trend.

3.3   Regression in R

Let's see how to fit a regression line in **R**. The data appears in a file, and printing it gives output similar to Output 2.7. In this example, each line represents the data on one infant. The columns represent the items or variables measured on each baby. There are 100 infants represented here, so we only include a few of the first and last of these. A short **R** program to plot the (x, y) values in Fig. 3.1, and find the least-squares slope and intercept, is given in Output 3.1.

The lm procedure does the actual fitting of the regression model. We assign the value and all of the output of the lm program to the variable reg. This allows us to extract the slope, intercept, and other useful information, as we will see.

The code wt~length specifies the model we are fitting: wt from length. Specifically, the dependent y variable (birth weight in this case) is on the left side of the equals sign, and the explanatory x variable (length, in this example) is listed on the right. There is no need to tell **R** to include an intercept, because this is the default.

Let's concentrate on just the portion of Output 3.1 produced by summary(reg). There is a summary of data about the residuals from this regression: minimum, maximum, the quartiles, and the median. In Chapter 4 we will examine residuals in more detail.

Output 3.1 includes information about the estimated regression line. This includes the least-squares estimates of the intercept ($\hat{\alpha} = -1171.253$) and slope ($\hat{\beta} = 61.654$). Exercise 3.3 asks you to interpret these values.

Both estimated parameters are associated with their respective standard errors. The ratio of the parameter estimate divided by its standard error is listed under the label t value. You should verify this is indeed the case. This statistic is used to test the null hypothesis that the underlying parameter being estimated has a population value of zero.

The rightmost column provides a p-value to test the statistical significance of this null hypothesis. In Output 3.1 these two p-values provide very strong evidence both the population slope and the intercept are nonzero.

Output 3.1 **R** program to compute a linear regression and produce Fig. 3.1.

```
> plot(birthwt$length, birthwt$wt, xlab = "Length",
     ylab = "Weight")          # plot length * weight in scatter plot
>
> reg <- lm(wt ~ length, data = birthwt) # fit the regression line
>
> lr <- c(25, 50)                  # range of length values in the plot
> y <- reg$coefficients[1] + reg$coefficients[2] * lr
> lines(lr, y, type = "l")         # add the line to the plot figure
> summary(lm)                      # print summary information

Call:
lm(formula = wt ~ length, data = birthwt)

Residuals:
    Min      1Q  Median      3Q     Max
-303.33 -113.71   -8.24   81.31  641.63

Coefficients:
              Estimate Std. Error t value Pr(>|t|)
(Intercept) -1171.253    163.469  -7.165 1.46e-10 ***
length         61.654      4.419  13.952  < 2e-16 ***
---
Signif. codes:  0 '***' 0.001 '**' 0.01 '*' 0.05 '.' 0.1 ' ' 1

Residual standard error: 157 on 98 degrees of freedom
Multiple R-squared:  0.6651,     Adjusted R-squared:  0.6617
F-statistic: 194.6 on 1 and 98 DF,  p-value: < 2.2e-16
```

Notice the statistical inference taking place in this statement: The estimated sample slope ($\hat{\beta}$) and intercept ($\hat{\alpha}$) are far enough from zero to lead us to conclude the population slope (β) and intercept (α) are also nonzero.

Why is this statement about statistical significance so important? A test of the slope is the primary reason for performing a linear regression in the first place. Our aim is to see if the x variable (length) has any value in explaining the outcome or dependent y variable, birth weight. If we concluded the regression slope was 0 then we would learn nothing about birth weight by knowing the baby's length. One of the most important tasks in proposing a statistical model is to demonstrate its value as an estimator of y. The demonstration of a statistically significant slope is one of the strongest pieces of evidence a data analyst can provide for the usefulness of a regression model. A test of significance of the intercept is usually not of interest to us, but see Exercise 3.3 for more details on the intercept in the present example.

Output 3.1 also demonstrates how you can capture the slope and intercept. These are given the name reg$coefficients. The fitted values $\hat{y}_i$ are obtained as reg$fitted.values. Recall these are the open circles in Fig. 3.2. The residuals r_i from the fitted regression can also be obtained from the output of lm. The most important diagnostic available to us is a plot of the residuals following a model fitting. This plot can disclose a variety of problems with a mathematical model of real data. These will be discussed in Section 4.4. To end this chapter, let us go over an example with what we have covered so far.

3.4 Statistics in the News: Future Healthcare Costs

The expansion of costs of US federal healthcare programs as a percentage of the total economy is of concern, and details of this can be seen in Fig. 3.3. The average age of the population is increasing in many industrialized nations. Older people consume more healthcare per person than their younger cohort.

The top line in this figure anticipates a huge rise in federal spending on healthcare programs. To many, this is cause for concern. Then again, the bottom line in this figure indicates a trend only slightly increasing. Many of the assumptions made here may prove invalid in the future. As times change, we can anticipate even more changes in future healthcare costs as well.

The estimates in this figure were based on assumptions which may or may not continue to be valid, even in the near future. Technology can rapidly change, and new medical discoveries may become commonplace. Congress could pass laws tomorrow, for example, changing systems of providing healthcare. All or none of this might

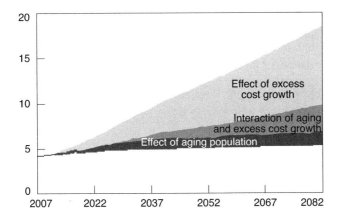

Figure 3.3 Projected healthcare cost estimates as a percentage of gross domestic product. *Source:* Congressional Budget Office.

happen, of course, and we cannot be sure when this might happen. The predictions made in this figure about events many years in the future could prove to be wildly inaccurate. Look at the wide range of possibilities between the three estimates.

> Extrapolate at your peril.

There is a danger of *extrapolating* beyond the data. The ability to fit regression lines does not give us license to describe events beyond the available data. There is no certainty the conditions generating the data will continue to hold. Linear regression can be abused in the wrong hands. Extrapolations, especially predictions about future events, should be made sparingly and need to be identified as such.

3.5   Exercises

3.1   Rewrite the two equations in (3.3) and (3.4) to convince yourself these really are two equations in two unknowns α and β. You will need to refer back to (3.1) to answer this question. If you are feeling very brave, try to solve these two equations for $\hat{\alpha}$ and $\hat{\beta}$.

3.2   Reread Section 2.7 and guess how many degrees of freedom are associated with the sum of squared residuals given in (3.2).

3.3   a.   The estimated slope in Output 3.1 is 61.65. Interpret this number. Specifically, what can you say about the average weights of two infants who differ by 1 cm in length?

b.   The estimated intercept in Output 3.1 is a large negative number. Is this cause for concern? How do we interpret the intercept in this model?

3.4   Fit the regression model explaining infant weight from gestational age. Provide a simple interpretation for the value of the slope in the fitted equation.

3.5   There may be some imprecision about the gestational age, but length can be measured fairly accurately. Use **R** to model gestational age from length. Why might this exercise be useful to a doctor?

3.6   The map in Fig. 3.4 shows drought conditions in the United States in the summer of 2020. The lack of rainfall was most acute in the west. Is this a map of the observed data, the expected mean values, or the residuals from the expected values? Which one of these three sets of values would be the best way to describe the weather conditions?

3.7   Examine the three weather maps in Fig. 1.1. Identify which of these represents the raw data, which is the expected, and which of these is the residual. Which of these is most useful to you? For example, is it more informative to know Florida was warm, Florida was expected to be warm, or Florida was colder than anticipated?

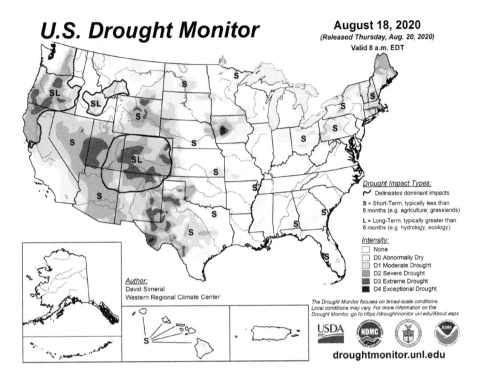

Figure 3.4 Map of drought conditions in the USA.
Source: US Drought Monitor, University of Lincoln-Nebraska.

Table 3.1 Average attendance at major league baseball games in 2019 season and population (in millions) of metropolitan area.

Team	Average attendance	Payroll in $M	Win %	Year-end rank Div.	Year-end rank League	Year-end rank Overall	Play-offs?	Pop.
Ariz Dbacks	26,364	123.9	0.52	2	7	13	N	4.948
Atlanta Braves	32,779	113.7	0.60	1	2	5	Y	6.020
Baltimore Orioles	16,146	72.7	0.33	5	14	29	N	2.800
⋮								
Wash. Nationals	27,899	161.8	0.57	2	3	9	Y	6.280

Source: The Baseball Cube and US Census.

3.8 A lot of sports-related data is collected but only recently has this been subjected to careful statistical methods. In this exercise we ask what determines attendance at major league baseball games? Table 3.1 lists the average attendance in the 2019 season for each team. Attendance was estimated by the number of tickets sold, not the numbers of fans who actually appeared at the games. Attendance is important to the local economy because fans will also visit restaurants and hotels in the vicinity of the stadium.

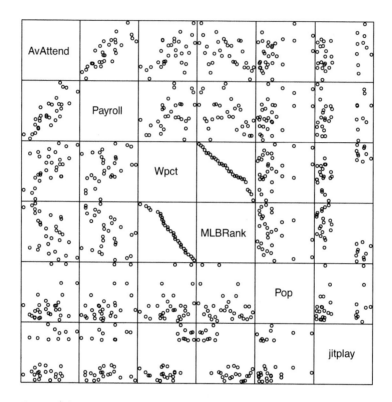

Figure 3.5 Scatter plot of baseball attendance data from Table 3.1.

Other related data include: team payroll (in $Million); percentage of games won in that season; season ending ranking by division, league, and overall; and whether or not the team appeared in the post-season playoffs. There were 30 teams divided into two leagues and each league was further divided into three divisions. We include 2019 Census population data for the metropolitan area as an estimate of the size of the potential audience.

A matrix scatter plot of some of the data is given in Fig. 3.5. The playoff values (Y/N) have been jittered for clarity. What relationships can you see here? Payroll appears closely related to average attendance. Does this suggest fans are more eager to see star athletes perform rather than have allegiance to the team? Are payroll and attendance related to the metropolitan population or are a few large markets standing apart from the others? Most of the team's revenue comes from broadcast rights. Larger markets can charge more for these although there is some revenue sharing to even out the imbalances between teams.

Winning percentage directly determines overall ranking and is closely related to whether or not the team appears in the playoffs. Can you suggest a way to compare average attendance values for teams with and without playoff appearances?

Table 3.2 Average weekly household expenditures (in £) on alcohol and tobacco in Great Britain.

Region	Alcohol	Tobacco
North	6.47	4.03
Yorkshire	6.13	3.76
Northeast	6.19	3.77
East Midlands	4.89	3.34
West Midlands	5.63	3.47
East Anglia	4.52	2.92
Southeast	5.89	3.20
Southwest	4.79	2.71
Wales	5.27	3.53
Scotland	6.08	4.51
Northern Ireland	4.02	4.56

3.9 Table 3.2 gives the average weekly household expenditures on alcohol and tobacco (measured in pounds sterling) for each of the regions of Great Britain as reported by official 1981 government statistics.[1]

Plot the data and fit a model explaining values of one expenditure from the other. Why would you think one of these variables should provide a good explanation for the values of the other?

From these data, can you conclude households consuming more tobacco are also those consuming more alcohol? The people who smoke may or may not be the same people who drink alcohol, for example. Such macro data as these tells us only about aggregate behavior and cannot always be used to explain data at the individual level.

3.5.1   Statistics in the News: Savings for Medicare

Rather than assign a fixed dollar amount for medical equipment and supplies, Medicare opened the prices for some of these items to competitive bidding in 2008. These changed the way in which Medicare reimburses suppliers for medical supplies. Some of these items (diabetic test strips and nutritional supplies) are consumed, and others (hospital beds and wound therapy pumps) are leased and reused (see Table 3.3).

Naturally, not everybody was pleased with this change. At the time, there was intense lobbying effort mounted against these changes by certain medical equipment suppliers.

---

[1] Available online at https://dasl.datadescription.com/datafile/tobacco-and-alcohol/.

Table 3.3 Changes in the way Medicare pays for certain medical supplies.

Type of equipment	Current price	New price	Percentage savings
Diabetic test strip, per 50	$36	$20	$43
CPAP respiratory device, per month	105	67	36
Enteral nutritional pump supplies, per day	12	9	30
Folding wheeled walker	112	78	30
Oxygen concentrator, per month	199	141	29
Hospital bed, per month	140	99	29
Standard power wheelchair	4024	3033	25
Wound therapy pump, per month	1716	1389	19
Power wheelchair with tilt system	8741	7530	

Source: Centers for Medicare and Medicaid Services.

Perform a linear regression, explaining the new price y using the current price x. Notice the largest percentage savings are generally associated with the least expensive items. Why do you think this might be the case? Which changes do you think might produce greater savings: a large percentage change in an item consumed in large amounts (such as the test strips) or a similar change in an expensive, specialized wheelchair only a few patients will need? Use linear regression to explain the percentage savings using the current price. Does this regression line have a useful interpretation?

3.5.2   Arsenic in Drinking Water

Arsenic is a potent poison, and ingesting or inhaling even small amounts can be fatal. It has been linked to a variety of different cancers as well. Long after death, arsenic is detectable in the hair of the victim, so cases of poisoning can be discovered years after the fact. In some places, arsenic is present in the ground water, slowly affecting those who drink from these sources. In the United States, municipal water sources are regularly tested, but private wells are not.

The data in Table 3.4 was part of an epidemiology study of drinking water in New Hampshire. Researchers from Dartmouth interviewed each of 21 residents who relied on private wells for much of their water for drinking or cooking. Each reported how much they relied on their private wells. (Household drinking and cooking use levels were coded as follows: 1, up to 1/4; 2, 1/4; 3, 1/2; 4, 3/5; and 5, over 3/4.) A sample of a toenail was taken from each resident and assayed for its arsenic content.

The arsenic levels in the water and toenails are measured in parts per million (ppm). A quick look at these values in Table 3.4 shows the toenail arsenic levels are all much higher than the water levels. This is consistent with the concentration of arsenic in the hair, long after ingestion.

Ideally, we might also want to know how long each resident had lived at their present address and relied on the well water. In Chapter 5 we see how to take into account the additional effects such as age, sex, and level of household well-water use.

Table 3.4 Arsenic levels in well water and toenails of 21 New Hampshire residents.

Age (years)	Sex 1 = M, 2 = F	Drinking use	Cooking use	Arsenic in water (ppm)	Arsenic in toenails (ppm)
44	2	5	5	0.00087	0.119
45	2	4	5	0.00021	0.118
44	1	5	5	0	0.099
66	2	3	5	0.00115	0.118
37	1	2	5	0	0.277
45	2	5	5	0	0.358
47	1	5	5	0.00013	0.080
38	2	4	5	0.00069	0.158
41	2	3	2	0.00039	0.310
49	2	4	5	0	0.105
72	2	5	5	0	0.073
45	2	1	5	0.046	0.832
53	1	5	5	0.0194	0.517
86	2	5	5	0.137	2.252
8	2	5	5	0.0214	0.851
32	2	5	5	0.0175	0.269
44	1	5	5	0.0764	0.433
63	2	5	5	0	0.141
42	1	5	5	0.0165	0.275
62	1	5	5	0.00012	0.135
36	1	5	5	0.0041	0.175

Source: Statlib.

For the present, use lm to fit a linear regression using well arsenic level to explain the toenail levels. Verify the fitted model is

$$\text{Toenail level} = 0.155 + 12.99 \times \text{Well-water level.}$$

Are you concerned the intercept is not zero? That is to say, with no exposure there should also be no arsenic in the toenail. Can you offer another explanation for the nonzero estimated intercept in this model?

We can fit a regression model in **R** with a zero intercept. The code to do this is as follows.

```
lm(toe ~ 0 + well, data = arsenic)
```

Run this program and verify the fitted model is

$$\text{Toenail level} = 14.87 \times \text{Well-water level.}$$

This model is interpreted as meaning toenail levels are *proportional to* well-water levels of arsenic. Does this model offer a better interpretation than the linear regression model with an intercept?

Why is the slope in the zero-intercept model (14.87) larger than the slope in the model with an estimated intercept (12.99)? It may help to plot the two fitted models in order to answer this question.

3.5.3   Dermatologists' Fees

Dermatologists treat disorders of the skin but may also perform cosmetic surgery. There is often a great divide between these two different roles. Some doctors will specialize in one or the other of these. Those who practice both cosmetic and medical surgery may have separate waiting rooms, appointment procedures, and treatment rooms for their patients, much as the airlines will segregate their first-class passengers from those paying to fly coach.

Medical procedures include the removal of moles and warts but also examination of cancerous and precancerous lesions. These are medically necessary procedures and are covered by Medicare and private insurance. Similarly, the reimbursement rates for these procedures are regulated by the amounts insurance will cover. Cosmetic procedures, on the other hand, are elective and are usually paid for out-of-pocket by the patient. Similarly, there is little oversight on how fees for cosmetic procedures are set. The data in Table 3.5 makes it very clear these different classes of procedures represent very different fees for the doctors.

Table 3.5 Dermatologists' fees for medical and cosmetic procedures.

Medical procedure	National average Medicare reimbursement	Estimated time spent by doctor
Abscess treatment	$96	15 to 20 min
New patient visit	62 to 91	5 to 30 min
Visit with skin cancer exam	60 to 90	5 to 20 min
Wart removal	89	up to 5 min
Mole biopsy	88	1 to 7 min
Psoriasis photo-therapy	75	20 s
Destruction of pre-cancerous lesion	67	30 s to 5 min

Cosmetic procedure	National average physician fee	
Laser skin resurfacing	$2418	30 to 40 min
Fat injection	1546	20 min
Chemical peel	718	5 to 10 min
Restylane injection	576	5 to 6 min
Laser vein treatment	462	5 min
Laser hair removal	387	2 to 5 min
Botox injection	380	1 to 10 min

Source: Inga Eitzey Practice Group, American Society for Aesthetic Plastic Surgery, Dr. Mark Knautz and Dr. Kenneth Mark.

We can easily see the difference in fees charged in this table. There is no need to resort to statistics to make the case these different types of procedures have a different fee schedule. Instead, let us see how the fee schedule is determined, separately for medical and cosmetic procedures. Table 3.5 includes a rough estimate of the amount of time the doctor will spend in performing each of several types of procedures. Is there evidence the fees charged are related to the time involved? Can we use linear regression to estimate the charge for a procedure based on the amount of time it takes to perform? There will be a separate regression line for medical and cosmetic procedures. Statisticians at insurance companies regularly use statistical methods such as these in order to determine reimbursement rates.

What assumptions do we need to make in order for this exercise to make sense? Do the various procedures (both medical and cosmetic) require additional equipment or drugs? This additional information would be useful in assigning a fee to a procedure. In this exercise we will need to assume all procedures have roughly the same overhead costs to the doctors. In cases where the time is given as a range, we might replace these with the midpoint or perhaps use the longest estimate of time as a worst-possible case.

What other information would you like to see before being able to estimate the fees charged? Table 3.5 does not include the relative frequencies of these various procedures. Should a commonly performed procedure, for example, be associated with a lower cost than one rarely performed, all other things being equal?

3.5.4 Breast Cancer Survival and Climate

It is well known some diseases have an environmental component. In a study of mortality rates in breast cancer, Table 3.6 provides the data for mean annual temperature in regions of Great Britain, Norway, and Sweden. Higher mortality rates translate into shorter survival times.

Fit a linear regression, estimating mortality rates from mean annual temperature. What is the equation of the fitted line? Look at a scatter plot of mortality and

Table 3.6 Breast cancer mortality rates in different countries.

Mortality rate	Mean annual temperature	Mortality rate	Mean annual temperature
102.5	51.3	104.5	49.9
100.4	50.0	95.9	49.2
87.0	48.5	95.0	47.8
88.6	47.3	89.2	45.1
78.9	46.3	84.6	42.1
81.7	44.2	72.2	43.5
65.1	42.3	68.1	40.2
67.3	31.8	52.5	34.0

Source: Lea (1965), based on public observation data from the UK Meteorological Office and other national databases.

temperature. Notice how two observations represent much colder climates than the remainder of the data. Do these two observations follow the general trend in the data? Is it reasonable to use your regression model to estimate mortality rates in the range of temperatures for which there is no data? Why do you think women in colder climates have better survival rates? What additional data would help you answer this question?

Is this an observational study or a randomized experiment? Reread Section 1.6 and compare these two different types of data. What are the similarities and differences between the IMF data and this breast cancer data in the way the data is collected and conclusions are drawn? Are we comfortable drawing conclusions from this study? What reservations did we have with drawing conclusions from the IMF data? Do you have the same reservations with using this data to draw any conclusions?

3.5.5   Cancer Mortality in Florida

If cancer mortality is related to climate in colder countries (Exercise 3.5.4), then is this statement also true in warmer climates? This idea was explored by Hart (2015), who examined mortality rates in Florida. Hart argued Florida was a good choice to explore this hypothesis because much of the state is at or near sea level so there would be no effect of exposure to cosmic radiation in addition to confounding effects of altitude and temperature.

We collected the data in Table 3.7 to test the hypothesis of a relation between climate and cancer mortality from government publications. Mean annual temperature (December 2019 to November 2020) was obtained from US National Centers for Environmental Information for each of the 67 counties in Florida. The temperature values and cancer rates shouldn't have varied much over the two-year difference. The cancer mortality rates are adjusted for differences in ages across the counties for the year 2008. In some counties, there were too few cancer cases to provide meaningful rates and these are listed as NA. **R** treats these values as missing.

Table 3.7 Mean temperature and age-adjusted cancer mortality rates in Florida counties.

County	Mean annual temperature	All cancers	Lung and bronchus	Prostate	Breast
Alachua	71.8	191.2	54.4	18.0	27.1
Baker	70.2	272.7	65.4	NA	NA
Bay	70.9	203.1	78.6	25.4	16.2
⋮			⋮		
Wakulla	71.0	190.3	66.9	NA	NA
Walton	69.6	158.3	48.1	28.4	25.2
Washington	70.0	222.9	82.8	NA	NA

Output 3.2 **R** program to read the Florida cancer mortality data, fit a linear regression, and produce Fig. 3.6.

```
> Fcan <- read.table(file = "Florida.txt", header = T, row.names = 1)
> Fcan[c(1 : 3, 65 : 67), ]     #  print first three and last three
           Temp   All LungB Prostate Breast
Alachua    71.8 191.2  54.4     18.0   27.1
Baker      70.2 272.7  65.4       NA     NA
Bay        70.9 203.1  78.6     25.4   16.2
Wakulla    71.0 190.3  66.9       NA     NA
Walton     69.6 158.3  48.1     28.4   25.2
Washington 70.0 222.9  82.8       NA     NA
>
> plot(Fcan$Temp, Fcan$All, xlab = "Mean annual temperature",
+      ylab = "Adjusted cancer rate", cex.lab = 1.25)
> Fcan[Fcan$All > 400, ]        #  Identify the outlier county
        Temp   All LungB Prostate Breast
Union 70.4 495.6 184.6       NA     NA
> text(71.7, 490, labels = "Union County")
>
> lm(All ~ Temp, data = Fcan)

Call:
lm(formula = All ~ Temp, data = Fcan)

Coefficients:
(Intercept)          Temp
     937.31        -10.24
```

Read the data into **R** and plot the different cancer rates by mean annual temperature. What do you see? There seems to be a strong relationship between climate and all cancers. This relationship is plotted in Fig. 3.6 using the **R** code given in Output 3.2. Does this relationship continue to hold for the three other specific cancers as well?

A notable outlier is identified in Fig. 3.6. Union County is the smallest county in the state and one of the poorest in the USA. This county includes a large prison. One third of the county residents are incarcerated in this facility. Prisoners from other facilities across the state needing healthcare are treated in the Union County prison hospital. Not only is this not a representative county but cancer cases diagnosed elsewhere are brought here from other counties.

Even if we exclude Union County from the plot in Fig. 3.6, does there still appear to be a relationship between climate and cancer mortality? Is there more information you would like to see? Florida is a popular destination for retirees, moving there from colder states and Canada. Many "snow birds" maintain two homes and reside

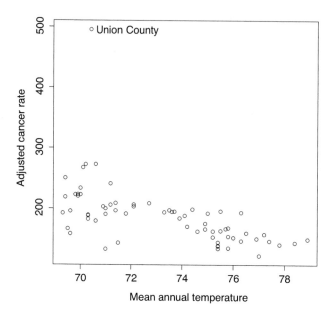

Figure 3.6 Adjusted cancer rates and mean annual temperature for Florida counties.

in Florida only during the winter months. What information would you like to see to address these effects on cancer mortality? As were saw in Exercise 3.5.4, do you have reservations about any conclusions to be drawn from this observational study?

3.5.6   Vital Rates

Government agencies go to great effort to collect vital information on the well-being of the population. Much of this data is made freely available to the public at no cost. Exercise 3.5.5 is an example of this. Another data set, selected from a large volume,[2] is given in Table 3.8 and presents the rates of the five leading causes of mortality in the United States from 1950 to 2004. In the year 1998 a definition was changed, and the data for that year is presented both with and without the adjustment.

Much can be learned by studying tables such as these. The good news is, there is a marked decrease in all-cause mortality. Within this statement, there have been changes in the specific causes of mortality. Use linear regression methods to show some rates such as heart disease and stroke have decreased over the years given in this table, but other rates such as those of cancer or respiratory diseases are flat or perhaps increasing.

Can you explain this finding? Despite a high level of funding for research, are we losing the war on cancer as some have claimed? Can you offer a different explanation?

---

[2] The document for 2007 is available online at www.cdc.gov/nchs/data/hus/hus07.pdf.

Table 3.8 Rates per 100,000 persons of the leading causes of death for all ages in the United States, 1950–2004.

Year	All-cause mortality	Heart disease	Cancer	Stroke	Respiratory diseases	Unintentional injury
1950	1446.0	586.8	193.9	180.7		78.0
1960	1339.2	559.0	193.9	177.9		62.3
1970	1222.6	492.7	198.6	147.7		60.1
1980	1039.1	412.1	207.9	96.2	28.3	46.4
1985	988.1	375.0	211.3	76.4	34.5	38.5
1990	938.7	321.8	216.0	65.3	37.2	36.3
1995	909.8	293.4	209.9	63.1	40.1	34.4
1996	894.1	285.7	206.7	62.5	40.6	34.5
1997	878.1	277.7	203.4	61.1	41.1	34.2
1998	870.6	271.3	200.7	59.3	41.8	34.5
1998*	870.6	267.4	202.1	62.8	43.8	35.6
1999	875.6	266.5	200.8	61.6	45.4	35.3
2000	869.0	257.6	199.6	60.9	44.2	34.9
2001	854.5	247.8	196.0	57.9	43.7	35.7
2002	845.3	240.8	193.5	56.2	43.5	36.9
2003	832.7	232.3	190.1	53.5	43.3	37.3
2004	800.8	217.0	185.8	50.0	41.1	37.7

*Adjusted because of a change in definitions.
Source: National Center for Health Statistics, *Health, United States, 2007.*

Perhaps the large drop in deaths due to heart disease is to blame for the lack of a decline in cancer rates. Is it possible an earlier cohort who would have died of heart disease before 1970 are replaced with a more recent population now living long enough to develop cancer?

4 Assessing the Regression

How do we know if our linear regression is any good? We can take the results from Output 3.1 and test the null hypothesis that the regression slope is zero. That is, could this apparent regression have happened by chance alone, if x and y were really unrelated? What tangible benefit can we claim for performing a linear regression? The analysis of variance described in this chapter allows us to quantify the information gained when we examine a linear regression model.

Is a straight line an appropriate summary for these data? Maybe there is a better explanation describing a curved relationship between x and y. Finally, if there are remarkable exceptions to the linear pattern, how can we identify these observations? This chapter and Chapter 5 use plots of the residual values to identify a large number of problems frequently arising when fitting mathematical models to real data.

4.1 Correlation

The correlation coefficient is a single-number summary expressing the utility of a linear regression. The correlation coefficient is a dimensionless number between -1 and $+1$. The slope and the correlation have the same positive or negative sign. This single number is used to convey the strength of a linear relationship, so values closer to -1 or $+1$ indicate greater fidelity to a straight-line relationship.

> The correlation measures the strength of a linear relationship.

The correlations in the low-birth-weight data are given in Output 4.1. The cor() function in **R** computes all possible pairwise correlations between columns in the data. The table of correlations is symmetric: values above and below the diagonal are the same. The correlation of x with y is the same as the correlation of y with x. Data values have perfect correlation with themselves, so the diagonal values are all equal to one. The values in this table should be compared with the matrix plot in Fig. 2.13.

The correlation is standardized so its value does not depend on the means or standard deviations of the x or y values. If we add or subtract the same values from the data (and thereby change the means), the correlation remains the same. If we multiply all the xs (or the ys) by some positive value, the correlation remains the same. If we multiply either the xs or the ys by a negative number, the sign of the correlation will reverse.

Output 4.1 Correlations in the low-birth-weight data.

```
> print(cor(birthwt), digits = 3)
            head    length    gage      wt    momage   pre.ecl
head       1.000    0.713    0.781   0.7988    0.132    0.1320
length     0.713    1.000    0.675   0.8156    0.218    0.1090
gage       0.781    0.675    1.000   0.6599    0.266    0.4120
wt         0.799    0.816    0.660   1.0000    0.155    0.0118
momage     0.132    0.218    0.266   0.1546    1.000    0.1141
pre.ecl    0.132    0.109    0.412   0.0118    0.114    1.0000
```

As with any oversimplification of a complex situation, the correlation coefficient has its benefits, but also its shortcomings. A variety of values of the correlation are illustrated in Fig. 4.1. Each of these separate graphs consists of 50 simulated (computer-generated) pairs of observations. A correlation of 0 in Fig. 4.1 (a) shows no indication of a linear relationship between the plotted variables. A correlation of 0.4 shows little or no relation. A correlation of either 0.8 or −0.9 indicates a rather strong linear trend. The sign of the correlation is the same as the sign of the slope.

It is possible to have a high correlation with little or no linear trend. The correlation of −0.9 in the example in Fig. 4.1 (d) is more the result of the small number of unusual individual observations than an indication of a true trend in the data. The big separated group in the upper-left corner is more representative of the population and exhibits no trend at all.

Similarly, a zero correlation does not indicate these measures are unrelated. In the example in Fig. 4.1 (f), we see the two variables have a very strong relationship, but it is not a *linear* relationship. The correlation coefficient is useful only to measure the strength of a linear relationship.

By looking at the plotted data in Fig. 4.1, we learn the correlation coefficient conveys an indication of a trend, but we still need to look at the scatter plot in order to understand the true nature of our data. Just as we say a picture is worth a thousand words, we could say a single number cannot possibly describe every situation we are likely to encounter. Despite these shortcomings, the correlation coefficient remains one of the most important summaries of the relationship between measurements on two variables.

The correlation coefficient is often expressed as its square and referred to as R^2 or *r-squared*. This definition is useful when we generalize linear regression to multivariate models in Chapter 5, where we consider models in which there are several explanatory variables. Just as with the correlation, the value of R^2 remains unchanged if we subject either of the two variables to a linear transformation. That is, we can add or subtract, multiply or divide (by a nonzero value) either the x or y variables, and the resulting values will have the same value of R^2.

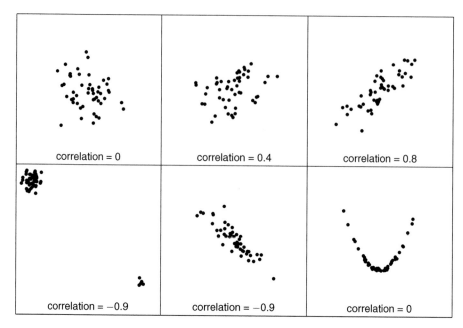

Figure 4.1 Simulated data sets illustrating different correlations.

4.2   Statistics in the News: Correlations of the Global Economy

In an article about investing,[1] Table 4.1 presents the correlations between returns in several foreign stock markets with those in the United States. The Standard and Poor's 500 (S&P 500) is a weighted average of prices of the stocks of the 500 largest US companies and is taken to represent almost all the US stock market. The table shows the correlation of each country's data with the S&P 500 over the previous five years. The MSCI EAFE Index, a weighted average of several countries' data, is also given here.

Some countries, notably Germany, France, and Spain, have stock markets closely following those in the United States. Such investments would not provide diversity and it would not be worth the additional risks of sending money overseas. Stock markets in India, Russia, and Japan, for example, have much lower correlation with those in the United States and would provide greater diversification.

Notice how a large amount of data has been reduced to a single number: the correlation. As we saw in Fig. 4.1, the correlation can be useful in some settings but may oversimplify more complex relationships. Domestic problems, such as a flood, may affect one country's economy but not others. Global changes in oil prices, for example, can affect many nations. The correlations in this table reflect all of these events, but do not offer an explanation or provide helpful details.

---

[1] Available online at www.nytimes.com/2007/06/03/business/yourmoney/03fund.html.

Table 4.1 The correlations between US and other foreign stock markets.

Country	Correlation with the S&P 500
Germany	0.89
France	0.88
Spain	0.85
MSCI EAFE	0.85
Britain	0.81
Italy	0.75
Mexico	0.74
Brazil	0.68
South Korea	0.67
Singapore	0.66
Hong Hong	0.55
China	0.53
India	0.43
Russia	0.35
Japan	0.29

Source: Standard & Poor's.

The article that accompanied this data concluded investments in Japanese stocks would provide a good counterbalance to those in Europe and the United States. An investment in Japan would not necessarily provide better returns, but might lower volatility in a portfolio. One market zigs while the other zags, so to speak. A small variability is reassuring when it comes to one's savings. Table 4.1 suggests a way in which investors could reduce the variance of their investment returns by diversifying across countries, but it does not explain how to increase the mean. (Which do you feel is more important: the mean rate of return, or the volatility experienced along the way?) The correlation is standardized, so it doesn't directly measure either of these.

Finally, notice there are no negative correlations in this data. It would be useful to know if there were stock markets moving in opposite directions, one rising while the others fell.

4.3   Analysis of Variance

Just as a statement from an accountant details how money was earned and spent, the analysis of variance (frequently abbreviated as ANOVA) is the statistician's table to explain, partition, and allocate variability in the data. To continue this analogy, variability is the currency of statistics. If all data always fell perfectly on a straight line, there would be no need for us to study statistics. Similarly, the ANOVA details the departure from a straight-line relationship.

What variability will we examine? Let us look back at Fig. 3.2 to see where the variability occurs. The residuals are defined in terms of the vertical differences so all of the variability occurs along the y axis. All of the variability occurs within the dependent variable we want to explain.

The variability of these values is measured by the following.

$$\text{Total sum of squares} = \sum (y_i - \bar{y})^2 \qquad (4.1)$$

This expression, divided by $n - 1$, is the familiar estimate of variance, s^2. We use s^2 to estimate the variance of y in the absence of any knowledge of an explanatory variable x. The expression for s^2 was given in (1.1). The analysis of variance allows us to quantify the benefit of knowing x and using it as an explanatory variable in a linear regression. This benefit is expressed as a reduction in the variability of the y values.

In the analysis of variance, the quantity in (4.1) is called the *total sum of squares*. In Section 2.7 we saw this expression is associated with $n - 1$ degrees of freedom. There are 100 observations in the low-birth-weight data, so this value is associated with 99 df.

The total sum of squares is the total amount of variability we have to work with. Ultimately we want to show how much of this variability is reduced by knowing x and how much is lost to random variability we cannot otherwise explain. Output 3.1 shows how **R** produces an ANOVA following a regression.

The *residual sum of squares* is just that: the sum of squared residuals, defined in (3.2), we want to minimize. The lm program finds the values of the slope and intercept minimizing this quantity. The residual sum of squares is the value at its minimum. This value is listed as Residuals in Output 4.2.

$$\text{Residual sum of squares} = \sum (\text{residual}_i)^2$$

There are 100 residuals in this example, but these are subject to two linear restrictions given by (3.3) and (3.4). Specifically, the residuals sum to 0 and are uncorrelated with the explanatory x values. These two restrictions result in a loss of 2 df, so Output 4.2 lists the residual sum of squares with $100 - 2 = 98$ df.

The residual sum of squares also goes by a variety of other names. Some books and computer programs will call this quantity the *error sum of squares*. Still other books and computer programs will call this the *unexplained variability* or the *unexplained sum of squares* because it represents the random noise left over after fitting the linear regression model.

The residuals represent departures from the model, and the model is fitted in a way making the residual sum of squares as small as possible. Intuitively, the residuals represent the part of the data not explained by the model; hence the name.

Output 4.2 Summary statistics and analysis of variance produced by the program in Output 3.1.

```
> reg <- lm(wt ~ length, data = birthwt) # fit the regression line
> summary(reg)                           # summary statistics of regression

Call:
lm(formula = wt ~ length, data = birthwt)

Residuals:
     Min       1Q   Median       3Q      Max
  -303.33  -113.71    -8.24    81.31   641.63

Coefficients:
             Estimate Std. Error t value Pr(>|t|)
(Intercept) -1171.253    163.469  -7.165 1.46e-10 ***
length         61.654      4.419  13.952  < 2e-16 ***
---
Signif. codes:  0 '***' 0.001 '**' 0.01 '*' 0.05 '.' 0.1 ' ' 1

Residual standard error: 157 on 98 degrees of freedom
Multiple R-squared:  0.6651, Adjusted R-squared:  0.6617
F-statistic: 194.6 on 1 and 98 DF,  p-value: < 2.2e-16

> anova(reg)                             # analysis of variance
Analysis of Variance Table

Response: wt
          Df  Sum Sq Mean Sq F value    Pr(>F)
length     1 4800035 4800035  194.65 < 2.2e-16 ***
Residuals 98 2416708   24660
---
Signif. codes:  0 '***' 0.001 '**' 0.01 '*' 0.05 '.' 0.1 ' ' 1
```

If the total sum of squares measures the whole amount of variability present in the data and the residual sums of squares is the unexplained portion of this, then the difference must be the part explained by the model. This difference is called the *model sum of squares* in Output 4.2. We can express this another way.

Total sum of squares = Model SS + Residual SS

In other words, the total amount of variability in the values (the y_i) we have can be decomposed into the sum of the amount explained by the model (knowing the xs), and the remainder is random noise or error.

Just as the sums of squares add up in this table, so do the degrees of freedom. The total sums of squares has $n - 1$ df and the residual sum of squares has $n - 2$ df. The degrees of freedom for the model sum of squares are equal to 1 in this example. When we build more complex models involving additional explanatory variables in Chapter 5, the model df will equal the number of explanatory variables in those models. For the time being, our model has only one explanatory variable, length, listed Output 4.2.

The R^2 has a useful interpretation in addition to being the squared correlation. The R^2 is also measures how much of the total variability is explained by the model. Specifically, the R^2 is

$$R^2 = \frac{\text{Model sum of squares}}{\text{Model sum of squares} + \text{Residual sum of squares}}.$$

We should look back at Output 4.2 and verify this is indeed the case. When R^2 is expressed in this fashion we see it also has the popular interpretation:

R^2 is the percent of total sum of squares explained by the model.

Other values in the ANOVA table are the mean squares. The values in the Mean Square column of Table 4.2 are obtained by dividing the sums of squares by their degrees of freedom.

The last entry for the ANOVA in Output 4.2 is the F value, which is calculated as

$$F = \frac{\text{MS(model)}}{\text{MS(error)}}.$$

The F statistic (sometimes called the F *ratio*) provides a statistical test of the contribution of the model in explaining the total variability of y. If we think of the model sum of squares as the explained variation and the error sum of squares as the unexplained part, we want this ratio to be large.

Another way to think about F is the signal-to-noise ratio. Ideally, we want a strong signal in the numerator relative to the noise component in the denominator. There are tables of the F statistic, but **R** will provide a p-value, so there is no real need to refer to tables.

The p-value of the F statistic provides a significance test of the null hypothesis that the slope of the regression model is zero. We have already seen such a test in Output 3.1. When there is only one explanatory variable, we have $t^2 = F$. In this particular example, we have $t = 13.952$ for the slope in Output 3.1 and $F = 194.65$ in Output 4.2. We can verify

$$13.952^2 = 194.65,$$

so here is another check on the relationships existing in the analysis of variance. In Chapter 5, when we talk about more than one x variable in the model, F provides a simultaneous test of whether *all* the slopes are zero.

The summary material in Output 4.2 provides a series of other useful statistics. These include the squared correlation coefficient ($R^2 = 0.6651$). The adjusted R^2 is described in Section 5.6 when we discuss multiple linear regression.

Perhaps the most useful number of all in this table is denoted by Residual standard error. In this table we can verify

$$\text{Residual standard error} = \sqrt{24660} = 157$$

is indeed the square root of the mean square for error in the analysis of variance.

This value represents the estimated standard deviation of the residuals. Recall the residuals represent the differences between the observed and expected values for our regression line. The residual standard error is the standard deviation or magnitude of this difference. This number tells us how far, on average, the observed data are to be expected from the fitted line. In the present example, if we wanted to estimate the weight of one of these infants from its length, the mean would be the fitted value on the regression line for the specified length and the standard deviation is estimated as 157 g.

Of course there will be outliers and exceptions to the rule, but if we assume observations are normally distributed about the regression line, then we can create an estimate of the standard deviation of that normal distribution. This brings us to the assumptions we make about the linear regression model which are described in the following section.

4.4   Model Assumptions and Residual Plots

The computer can always calculate whatever you ask it to, but it cannot judge the validity or appropriateness of the methods used. The p-value for the F statistic in the analysis of variance represents a calculation made by a machine not knowing anything about how your data was obtained or whether the model is appropriate. In order for the model to explain accurately the data and for your p-value to represent a meaningful test of the null hypothesis, we need to make some assumptions about the data.

Many diagnostics about the regression model can be derived using plots of the residuals of the fitted model. The residuals can easily be obtained and examined, but the crucial concept is these are sampled from a larger, unobservable population. In Section 1.1 we make this distinction between sampled data and the larger population. As with all statistical inference, a sample (in this case, of residuals) is used to infer properties of a much larger population. This population is referred to as the *error distribution*. The residuals are an observed sample of errors.

The model assumptions are expressed in terms of the error distribution. These are as follows.

1. Errors are independent.
2. Errors have constant variance.
3. Errors have mean zero.
4. Errors follow a normal distribution.

Think of the regression model as a series of normal distributions centered along the regression line. Figure 4.2 will help you visualize this. At any given value of x, there is a y value sampled from the normal distribution whose mean is equal to $\alpha + \beta x$. The standard deviation of this regression line is estimated by the residual standard error, described in the previous section.

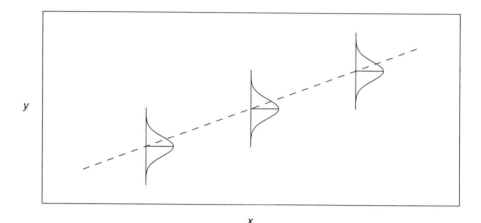

Figure 4.2 The idealized regression model is a series of normal distributions centered along the regression line.

All the assumptions we make about the model concern the errors. We cannot observe the errors: we only have a sample of residuals from the population. The most important message, then, is we must take the residuals very seriously. We cannot abrogate our responsibility and ask for a statistical test of these assumptions to let us off the hook. One of the most important tools available to us is to do the following.

> Plot and examine the residuals for your model.

This one simple technique is, by far, the most powerful yet simple way to diagnose many of the problems existing in a regression model. The true difficulty will be for the user of these methods to verify the assumptions are met. The computer cannot do this for us. We need to examine these plots and try to infer whether or not the model is appropriate. The residual values are typically plotted on the vertical axis, and the horizontal axis might be either the explanatory value x or the estimated value $\hat{y}$.

Figure 4.3 presents a set of four problems in data analysis arising when we perform a linear regression. In most cases the residual plot will magnify the problem and make it more easily apparent and diagnosed. In Fig. 4.3 (a) we see the relationship between x and y is not a straight line. The residual plot magnifies the curvature in the relationship. These residuals clearly do not represent white noise, and the curved trend is clear in the right-hand plot in (a).

In the second pair of plots, Fig. 4.3 (b), we see an example of the violation of the assumption of constant variance. The residual plot has a funnel shape, indicating increasing variability with larger values of x. The regression line will be overly influenced by the observations with larger variability because these observations tend to appear farther away from the line. As a result, we see the linear model has a poor fit for smaller values of x on the left-hand side of (b) where the model is most appropriate.

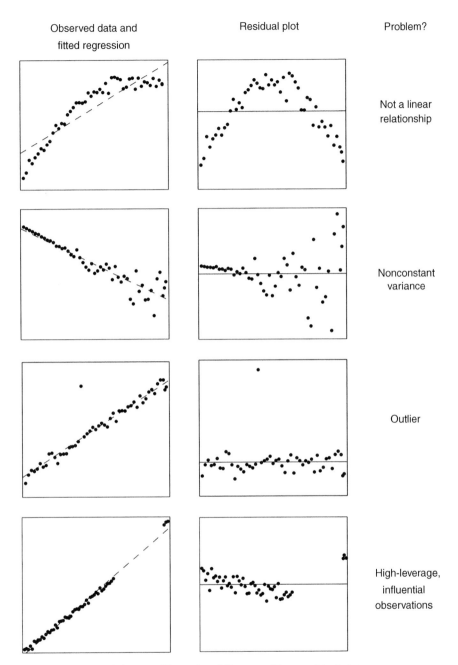

Figure 4.3 Simulated data sets illustrating different problems residual plots may uncover.

An outlier is an observation failing to follow the form of the model for any of a variety of reasons. Sometimes outliers are simply errors in coding of the data, such as a pair of reversed digits. These can be replaced, or the observation can be deleted. In other settings the outliers may have tremendous value to us.

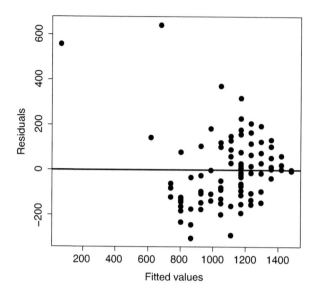

Figure 4.4 Residuals for low-birth-weight babies.

As an example, in the 2000 US presidential election, the third-party candidate, Patrick Buchanan, received more votes in one Florida county than in the entire remainder of the country combined. The election results were presented before the US Supreme Court to decide whether these votes were valid or not.

An outlier can sometimes provide deeper insight into what our data really represents. It is up to us to decide whether or not our outliers are important, but they should be identified in any case (see Fig. 4.3 (c)).

The pair of plots in Fig. 4.3 (d) illustrate the effect of influential observations. These are not necessarily far from the regression line, but their unusual explanatory values cause them to exert a large influence on the fitted value of the estimated slope and intercept. We sometimes say such observations have high leverage. Measures of leverage and influence are discussed in Chapter 5.

Notice the downward-sloping trend in the group of observations on the left side of the residual plot of Fig. 4.3 (d). The high-leverage points on the right side pull the regression line toward themselves. This makes the remaining observations appear to be ill fitted by the model.

An example of the residuals from the low-birth-weight infants data of Section 3.1 appears in Fig. 4.4. In **R** we can fit a regression and plot residuals to produce this figure with the following lines.

```
reg <- lm(wt ~ length, data = birthwt)
plot(reg$fitted.values, reg$residuals, xlab = "Fitted values",
     ylab = "Residuals", pch = 19)
lines(x = c(00, 1600), y = c(0,0))  # draw horizontal axis line
```

Exercise 4.6 asks you to look at this plot and identify unusual or remarkable obser-vations. Exercise 4.1 asks you to examine the four model assumptions described in this section for a data set appearing in the news.

4.5   Exercises

4.1   Figure 4.5 is a graph of US airline profits since 2001, plotted by year. Suppose we were to produce a linear regression on profit using the year as the explanatory variable. Look at the four important assumptions in Section 4.4. Which of these model assumptions are valid and which are violated when we perform this linear regression?

4.2   What is the largest correlation we can achieve with exactly three pairs of obser-vations? Draw a scatter plot to show how this can be achieved. Similarly, can a cor-relation of exactly 0 be achieved with three pairs of observations? What might this scatter plot look like?

4.3   Suppose I found the correlation between x and y. If I add 5 to all of the x values, what is the new correlation between x and y? If I multiply all the y values by 3, what is the new correlation? If I multiply all the values of x by -2, what is the new correlation between x and y?

4.4   I prepared an analysis of variance for homework, but my dog ate it. All that is left is given in Table 4.2. Can you fill in the missing parts?

4.5   Look back at the arsenic data examined in Exercise 3.5.2. Examine the residuals for this fitted regression and compare your plot to those in Fig. 4.3. Identify the

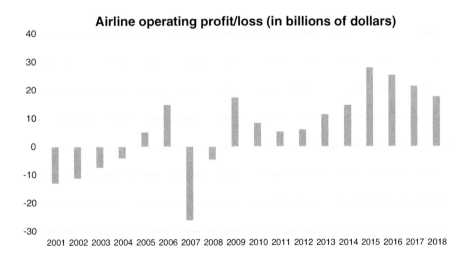

Figure 4.5 Airline profits 2001–2018.
Source: Bureau of Transportation Statistics.

Table 4.2 Part of the output for Exercise 4.4.

Source	df	Sum of squares	Mean square	F value
Model	1			4.0
Residual			8.0	
Total	21			

individual with the highest arsenic exposure. Is this observation influential in the regression model? What happens to the fitted regression coefficients when this one individual is deleted and the model is refitted?

4.6 a. Look at the low-birth-weight data on infants from Chapter 3. The residuals from the regression in Fig. 3.1 are given in Fig. 4.4. What do you learn by looking at this figure? Can you identify outliers or highly influential observations? The variability of the residuals seems to decrease with the fitted value. Why does this appear to be the case? Remember what it means for an infant to have a low birth weight.

   b. Fit some other regression models to the low-birth-weight data. Draw some graphs of observed values and the residuals from your regression. Comment on what you see. See if you can find outliers and or influential observations. Identify the equation of your linear regression. Cite statistical measures of significance levels.

   Why did you choose the explanatory x and response y variables you did? Is linear regression appropriate for this pair of values in the data set? Are there other variables you would like to know about not given here? What additional knowledge do you have about infants you can use to provide a better understanding of the examination of this data?

4.7 Fit a regression model to the baseball attendance data in Table 3.1. Specifically, show how average attendance is directly related to the teams' payrolls. Examine the residuals from this regression model. Do these reveal any departures from the assumptions we make for regression models?

4.5.1   Food Imports

Following reports of tainted pet food, seafood, toothpaste, and pharmaceutical additives from China, the data in Table 4.3 appeared,[2] demonstrating food shipments are refused by US customs officials from other countries as well. Common sense indicates the number of shipments refused should be related to the total number of shipments. The numbers of shipments are not provided, but instead the figure gives the total value of all food imports for each of the countries listed.

---

[2] Available online at www.nytimes.com/2007/07/12/business/12imports.html.

Table 4.3 Food import shipments refused at the border by the FDA. Those countries with the largest number of refusals are listed.

Country	Number of shipments refused	Frequency of most common refusal	Total value food imports
India	1763	256	$1.2B
Mexico	1480	385	9.8
China	1368	287	3.8
Dominican Republic	828	789	0.3
Denmark	543	85	0.4
Vietnam	553	118	1.1
Japan	508	143	0.5
Italy	482	138	2.9
Indonesia	460	122	1.5

Plot the value of the total food imports (as the explanatory variable x) against the number of shipments refused (y). What do you see? Does the slope go in the direction you expected it to? Can you provide an explanation for this?

Notice the very large influence in this graph of the total food imports from Mexico. The total value of these imports is about as great as all of the other listed countries' imports combined. Why do you think this may be the case?

Relatively few shipments from Mexico are refused in comparison to other countries. What do you think is the reason for this? Look at the most frequent reasons given for food refused from Japan, Denmark, and Italy to see if this may be the case. These countries also export relatively small amounts of food to the United States.

Fit the linear regression with all of the data and then again excluding Mexico. Is the fitted model different? Comment on the change in correlation and the statistical significance in the F-ratio.

The total import value data covers the calendar year 2006 but does not exactly coincide with the time period for the food shipment refusal data. What additional data would you need to see if imports from China were being given greater scrutiny following news reports? What additional information would you need in order to tell if food imports from all source countries were being examined more closely following the news?

4.5.2 US Homicide Rates

Violence is recognized as a public health problem. Reports of violent crime are shocking and can serve different purposes depending on who is citing the statistics.

The figures in Table 4.4 were compiled by the Congressional Research Service when several mass shootings were followed by calls for stronger gun control measures. Table 4.4 lists the number of US murders and the numbers of these related to firearms. Both of these figures are also adjusted to rates per 100,000 persons to reflect changes in the population.

Table 4.4 US murder and firearm rates by year.

Year	Murder victims Number	Murder victims per 10^5	Firearm victims Number	Firearm victims per 10^5
1993	24,526	9.5	17,073	6.6
1994	23,326	9.0	16,333	6.3
1995	21,606	8.2	14,727	5.6
1996	19,645	7.4	13,261	5.0
1997	18,208	6.8	12,335	4.6
1998	16,974	6.3	11,006	4.1
1999	15,522	5.7	10,117	3.7
2000	15,586	5.5	10,203	3.6
2001	16,037	5.6	10,139	3.6
2002	16,229	5.6	10,841	3.8
2003	16,528	5.7	11,037	3.8
2004	16,148	5.5	10,665	3.6
2005	16,740	5.6	11,363	3.8
2006	17,309	5.8	11,731	3.9
2007	17,128	5.7	11,631	3.9
2008	16,645	5.4	11,029	3.6
2009	15,399	5.0	10,301	3.4
2010	14,722	4.8	9,812	3.2
2011	14,612	4.7	9,903	3.2

Source: Congressional Research Service
Nov. 14, 2012. 7-5700: RL32842.

Draw some graphs and explain any trends you see. Use Year as the explanatory variable and show if these trends have statistical significance. Create a new variable to examine the percent firearm murders make of all murders. How does this fraction change over the years covered in this table?

4.5.3　Statistics in the News: Women Managers

We hear about the "glass ceiling" preventing women from being promoted to the ranks of management when compared to rates for men. The data in Table 4.5 compares the promotion rates in 10 different countries. For each country we have the percentages of women employed as managers in the years 1985 and 2005. The accompanying article[3] points out although Japan has passed several antidiscrimination laws, these laws are rarely enforced, and there is a cultural reluctance to initiate lawsuits. There has also been little change in South Korea, but the other Asian nations of Singapore and Malaysia have made large advances in promoting women to management positions.

---

[3] www.reuters.com/article/us-japan-companies-women/women-in-management-at-japan-firms-still-a-rarity-reuters-poll-idUSKCN1LT3GF.

Table 4.5 Percentage of management jobs held by women in 1985 and 2005.

Country	Percent of female managers	
	in 1985	in 2005
Philippines	21.9	57.8
United States	35.6	42.5
Germany	25.8	37.3
Australia	17.6	37.3
Britain	32.9	34.5
Norway	22.0	30.5
Singapore	12.0	25.9
Malaysia	8.7	23.2
Japan	6.6	10.1
South Korea	3.7	7.8

Source: World Economic Forum.

Use linear regression to explain the 2005 rates in terms of the 1985 rates. Plot the raw data. Is there evidence the variance is not constant? Explain why this might be the case. Examine the fitted regression coefficients and explain these values in terms of the original data.

Suppose we wanted to examine the percentage change in these rates. Construct a new variable defined as the 2005 rate divided by the 1985 rate. Perform a linear regression to explain this new variable from the 1985 rate. Notice the slope is negative. Does this mean those countries with the lowest 1985 rates tended to have the greatest percentage increase in women managers? Can you provide a different interpretation of this regression slope?

4.5.4   Statistics is More Than Just Numbers

Francis J. Anscombe[4] was the founder of the Statistics Department at Yale University. He created the four data sets given in Table 4.6. There is so much to learn by examining these. If you examine only the statistics from the computer output, you might be led to think these four were the same data.

In this exercise, pick any two of these four data sets and see how similar the computed numbers appear when you regress y on x. Find means and standard deviations in **R**. Which summary statistical measures are the same for the pair of data sets you choose? How different are the two ANOVAs? If you are unsure, try looking at a third data set. In what ways are the data sets different? You might begin, for example, by noting the first three data sets all have identical values for their x variable.

When you are done, look at the scatter plot of x and y values for the data sets you examined. Note how very different these are. Describe each data set in a sentence or

---

[4] Francis John Anscombe (1918–2001), British statistician.

Table 4.6 The four data sets from Anscombe (1973), listed as (x,y) pairs.

First data set							
10	8.04	8	6.95	13	7.58	9	8.81
11	8.33	14	9.96	6	7.24	4	4.26
12	10.84	7	4.82	5	5.68		

Second data set							
10	9.14	8	8.14	13	8.74	9	8.77
11	9.26	14	8.10	6	6.13	4	3.10
12	9.13	7	7.26	5	4.74		

Third data set							
10	7.46	8	6.77	13	12.74	9	7.11
11	7.81	14	8.84	6	6.08	4	5.39
12	8.15	7	6.42	5	5.73		

Fourth data set							
8	6.58	8	5.76	8	7.71	8	8.84
8	8.47	8	7.04	8	5.25	8	5.56
8	7.91	8	6.89	19	12.50		

Available as anscombe in **R**.

two. Notice how the summary statistics fail to tell us what the data actually is. Which description is more meaningful: the graph or the summary statistics? Which would you rather have?

The conclusion of this exercise is an important lesson.

> Statistics is much more than formulas and numbers.

It is possible to summarize data in any number of ways and still miss the point. You might think the mean and standard deviation contain just about all you need to know about your data, and if you do, you could be way off the mark. A correlation could represent a wide variety of different situations. We saw this in the examples of Fig. 4.1. You might reread the example appearing in Section 1.6 to see how statistical methods can be carefully applied and still yield absurd conclusions.

5 Multiple Regression and Diagnostics

We often have several possible explanatory variables to help us model an outcome variable. Some of these have more explanatory value than others, some may be redundant, and others may be totally useless.

Multivariate models bring a new set of challenges for modeling data. Nevertheless, there are rewards for our efforts: we are often able to summarize a large amount of data in a succinct fashion; interesting relationships will appear; but unfortunately, exceptions to the rule may also appear. Ultimately, we gain a deeper understanding of the world through the observed data.

5.1 Example: Maximum January Temperatures

The data set listed in Table 5.1 provides the maximum January temperature for many US cities. Also given are latitude (degrees North from the equator); longitude (degrees East/West); and altitude above sea level in feet. A small regression program is given in Output 5.1.

Let's start by comparing the January data in Table 5.1 with the birth-weight data in Output 2.7. One of the biggest differences is the inclusion of *text* in the temperature data, namely the city names. To read text fields in **R** we need to prepare our data carefully and then correctly specify the appropriate **R** code. Always print the data after reading it. It is useful to print a few lines from the beginning as well as the end and compare these with the original data in the file.

The regression model fitted by the program in Output 5.1 is

$$\text{maxt} = \alpha + \beta_1 \text{lat} + \beta_2 \text{long} + \beta_3 \text{alt} + \text{error}. \tag{5.1}$$

The model specifies the maximum January temperature is linearly related to each of latitude, longitude, and altitude, separately. The lm program estimates the intercept α and each of the regression slopes β_1, β_2, and β_3. We interpret this model to mean the maximum January temperature is the sum of the individual effects of latitude, longitude, and altitude. There is an intercept (α) and three regression slopes needed to be estimated. In such a model we sometimes say temperature is *corrected* for the separate effects of these three explanatory variables.

Table 5.1 Maximum January temperature (*T*, in degrees Fahrenheit), latitude (Lat), longitude (Long), altitude in feet above sea level (Alt), and the name for the some of the largest US cities.

T	Lat	Long	Alt	Name	*T*	Lat	Long	Alt	Name
61	30	88	5	Mobile AL	59	32	86	160	Montgomery AL
30	58	134	50	Juneau AK	64	33	112	1090	Phoenix AZ
51	34	92	286	Little Rock AR	65	34	118	340	Los Angeles CA
⋮									
31	47	117	1890	Spokane WA	26	43	89	860	Madison WI
28	43	87	635	Milwaukee WI	37	41	104	6100	Cheyenne WY
81	18	66	35	San Juan PR					

Data from Mosteller and Tukey (1977, pp. 73–4), with corrections.

In the `lm` function in Output 5.1 we express the model as

$$\texttt{MJtemp \textasciitilde{} Lat + Long + Alt}$$

putting the dependent variable we wish to explain on the left of the ˜ sign and provide a list of the explanatory variables on the right. The **R** programming is then no more difficult than what we saw in Chapter 3. Output 5.1 lists (among other things) estimates for the intercept (α) and each of the three regression coefficients (βs) along with their standard errors.

Northern cities are colder than most, as are cities at high altitudes. We should not be surprised to see the corresponding negative estimated slopes in Output 5.1 because these represent negative correlations.

Let us interpret some of the information given in Output 5.1. The estimated regression coefficient for latitude (-1.95981), is negative. We can intuit for every degree North of the equator, the temperature drops by almost 2 degrees Fahrenheit. This estimate is more than 18 times its estimated standard error (0.10481) so latitude has a huge effect in explaining the different temperatures of the various cities. The estimated regression coefficient for longitude is positive but its value is not statistically different from zero.

The `Coefficients` paragraph in the output of `lm` provides an estimated value, a standard error, and a test of statistical significance for each term in the model. The test of significance tests the null hypothesis the underlying population parameter is zero. The F-statistic provides a significance test of the null hypothesis: all of the regression slopes are zero in the population.

Altitude also plays a large role in explaining the different temperatures. Cities at higher altitudes are colder; hence the negative estimated regression coefficient. For every 1000 feet above sea level, the estimated temperature drops 1.64 degrees. The estimated intercept ($\hat{a}$) in this table and other analyses of these data are described in Exercise 5.7.2.

Output 5.1 A program for the January temperature data.

```
> Jan <- read.table(file = "Jan.txt", sep = "\t",
+                        header = T, row.names = 5)
> (leng <- dim(Jan)[1])              # number of rows
[1] 61
> Jan[1:3, ]                         # print first three rows
                MJtemp Lat Long Alt
Mobile AL           61  30   88   5
Montgomery AL       59  32   86 160
Juneau AK           30  58  134  50
> Jan[(leng-2) : leng, ]             # print last three rows
                MJtemp Lat Long  Alt
Milwaukee WI        28  43   87  635
Cheyenne WY         37  41  104 6100
San Juan PR         81  18   66   35
>
> reg <- lm(MJtemp ~ Lat + Long + Alt, data = Jan)
> summary(reg)

Call:
lm(formula = MJtemp ~ Lat + Long + Alt, data = Jan)

Residuals:
     Min       1Q   Median       3Q      Max
-13.7292  -2.9324   0.8911   3.0289  14.6619

Coefficients:
              Estimate Std. Error t value Pr(>|t|)
(Intercept)  1.009e+02  5.193e+00  19.437  < 2e-16 ***
Lat         -1.960e+00  1.048e-01 -18.699  < 2e-16 ***
Long         2.100e-01  4.129e-02   5.086 4.25e-06 ***
Alt         -1.643e-03  5.179e-04  -3.172  0.00244 **
---
Signif. codes:  0 '***' 0.001 '**' 0.01 '*' 0.05 '.' 0.1 ' ' 1

Residual standard error: 5.364 on 57 degrees of freedom
Multiple R-squared:  0.872, Adjusted R-squared:  0.8652
F-statistic: 129.4 on 3 and 57 DF,  p-value: < 2.2e-16
```

Estimates of the regression coefficients $(\alpha, \beta_1, \beta_2, \beta_3)$ for the model in (5.1) are obtained by **R** using least squares. Specifically, these are obtained by making the sum of squared errors as small as possible. This approach for estimating regression parameters was covered in Section 3.2 for a model with a single explanatory variable. The same approach is followed here in multiple regression models, except **R** will minimize an expression similar to (3.2) with respect to each of the regression slopes.

The output of `lm` in multiple regression includes the analysis of individual regression terms given in Output 5.1 and can be compared to the output given in Output 4.2. The largest difference we see is the model sums of squares will have 1 df for every regression slope appearing in the model. As with simple linear regression, the sums of squares and df will add up just as in Exercise 4.4. The mean squares are again defined as sums of squares divided by their degrees of freedom.

Here are some things to think about as we proceed. What about northern cities at high altitude? Are their January temperatures the sum of their parts or is there a synergy? Synergy occurs when two factors combine to produce a greater effect than either one individually, working together like a well-practiced team. Think of it as a situation in which $1 + 1 = 3$. We address synergy in Section 6.3. The present chapter describes several measures of influence and other diagnostic measures. Before we get to these topics, we look at a variety of graphical displays for multivariate data such as these.

5.2   Graphical Displays of Multivariate Data

Let us examine two popular methods for graphically displaying the data. A moment's reflection will reveal the display of multivariate data is a challenging task: it is very difficult to display several different kinds of information simultaneously on a two-dimensional piece of paper. A bit of creativity has been needed and used to create these displays. This section introduces a few of these methods.

The scatter plot is well known to the reader. The display in Fig. 5.1 provides a matrix of scatter plots for every pair of variables in the linear regression model. The diagonal of this display lists the names of the variables and the range of their values. Each plot is provided twice as a pair of graphs transposed of each other. Specifically, in the first row, the maximum temperature is the vertical axis and is plotted against all other variables. In the first column, the maximum temperature is again plotted against all other variables, but now along the horizontal axis. This figure is produced by `plot(Jan)`. The `plot` function is a useful procedure in **R** with many available options.

When we look at Fig. 5.1, we see the only linear relationship is between temperature and latitude, given in the two plots in the upper-left corner of this figure. These relationships are negatively correlated because more northerly cities are generally colder.

These plots also reveal altitude is not well correlated with any of the other variables. The plots in the last row and column show plots of altitude against all other variables. Most of the US cities are located at or near sea level, so many altitude values are small. There are only a few high-altitude cities with values much larger than others.

The bubble plot of Fig. 5.2 provides a three-dimensional map of the US cities. Values of latitude and longitude locate the cities in a familiar manner. The diameters

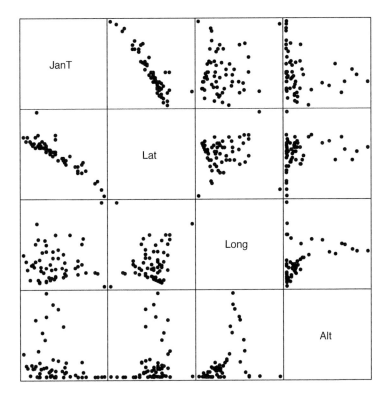

Figure 5.1 Matrix scatter plot of the January temperature data.

of the circles are proportional to their altitude. The resulting figure is called a `bubble plot` because of its overall appearance. In addition to the familiar map of the United States, we also see the largest altitudes are in the West, medium altitudes occur in the Midwest, and coastal cities, as their name implies, are situated at sea level.

This plot is produced in **R** using the code in Output 5.2. The variable `longe` is longitude measured in degrees East. The `cex =` option in the `plot` statement controls the sizes of the bubbles. Three cities with extreme longitude are identified by sorting these values then locating the smallest and two largest. The `match` command identifies the indexes of these three cities. These indexes are assigned to the variable `ext`. The names of three remarkable cities have been added to this figure using the `text` feature.

The graphical display of data, and more generally information has come a long way. We could only provide two examples in this section. For additional reading, look into the series of books by Tufte (2011). Tufte describes the good and bad features of graphic displays and shows how to improve our presentations. At a deeper level, Wilkinson (2005) develops a new language to create graphical displays. These have been implemented in the `ggplot2` package in **R**.

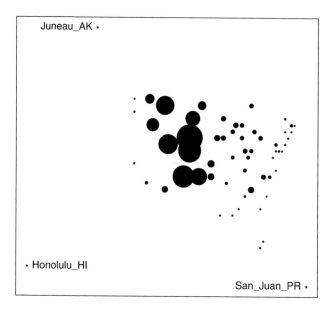

Figure 5.2 Bubble plot map of major US cities. Bubble sizes are related to altitude.

Output 5.2 R code to produce the bubble plot in Fig. 5.2.

```
Longe <- 180 - Jan$Long              # Longitude, east
Jan <- cbind(Jan, Longe)             # Append this column
Jan[1:5, ]                           # Check to see if this worked

n <- dim(Jan)[1]                     # number of cities
plot(Jan$Longe, Jan$Lat, lwd = 2, xaxt = "n", xlab = "",
     yaxt = "n", ylab = "", cex = 0.5 + Jan$Alt / 1000)
ext <- match(sort(Jan$Long)[c(1, n, n-1)],
             Jan$Long)               # identify index of 3 extreme cities
text(Jan$Longe[ext], Jan$Lat[ext],   # label three extreme cities
     labels = row.names(Jan)[ext], pos = c(2, 4, 2))
```

5.3   Leverage and the Hat Matrix Diagonal

In Section 4.4 we saw that the most important diagnostic tool available to us is the residual plot. By looking at the differences between the observed values of the dependent variable y and those $\hat{y}$ estimated by the model, we can often identify outliers representing obvious deviations from the model in explaining the entire data set. In contrast to the examination of residuals, the measures described in this section identify observations said to have *high leverage* because they are outliers in terms of their explanatory x variables.

For an example of leverage, let us look back at Fig. 4.3. The pair of plots in Fig. 4.3 (d) exemplify a data set in which a small number of points with unusual explanatory x values have a large leverage on the fitted model. If the problem is due to the y value then we attribute this to outliers or observations failing to follow the model. Outliers are usually identified by plotting the residuals. Leverage points, however, are due to unusual values of the explanatory variables, and these may be more difficult to identify in multiple linear regression.

If we had only one explanatory variable, a simple plot of the data would reveal high-leverage observations because of their extreme values. Look back at the low-birth-weight infant data in Fig. 3.1. The residuals of that regression are given here as Fig. 5.3. Notice how one very short infant appears at the far left of this figure. The data on this one infant has a large effect: it pulls the fitted regression line toward itself, resulting in a line appearing to overestimate the weights of the other smallest infants in the data. For this reason, we say such an observation has a high amount of leverage because it is so far away from the other data values of the explanatory variable.

Why are high-leverage observations so difficult to identify? The problem with multivariate regression models is that a group of several explanatory variables may collectively have unusual values but may not be extreme in any one of them. For two weather-related examples, a chilly day (but not the coldest) along with a light drizzle (but not the heaviest rain) may result in an experience of the worst weather. As another example, the wind chill factor is a combined measure of cold and wind in which a

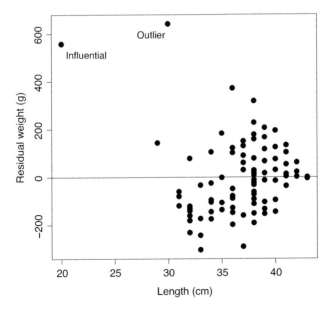

Figure 5.3 Residual plot of birth weight and length of 100 low-birth-weight infants. Two remarkable data points are identified.

particular temperature on a windy day feels equivalent to a much colder temperature without the wind. The weather feels extreme even though the temperature may not be unusually low.

The *hat matrix diagonal* is a popular method for describing leverage in multivariate regression. The mathematical form of the hat matrix is more than we need here, but we can express it in a simple form making it easier to remember. The hat matrix has the property

$$\text{Hat matrix} \times \text{Observed} = \text{Expected}.$$

That is, the hat matrix acts on the observed y values, collectively, and transforms these into the fitted or expected $\hat{y}$ values. Written another way, we have

$$\text{Hat} \times Y = \hat{Y}. \tag{5.2}$$

In this last expression we see the hat matrix "puts the hat on Y"; hence the name. This transformation is smooth in the sense each observed y value contributes to each fitted value, including its own. Ideally, we want this process to be uniform, where all of the observations are used equally to help estimate their own fitted values.

The diagonal of the hat matrix shows how much each individual observation contributes to its own fitted value. In the ideal situation, all observations would provide an equal amount to their own fitted values, along with some smaller amount of information about the others. Again, these should all be about the same amount for each observation in the data.

Observations contributing much more than others to their own fitted values are suspect and should be identified. In an extreme setting, an observation providing the information about its own fitted value is not really following the model at all. For this to happen, the values of the explanatory variables of this observation will have to be very unusual.

What is not obvious from expression (5.2) is that the hat matrix depends only on the explanatory values and not on the dependent y values. The interpretation, then, is that the hat matrix is a measure of leverage among the independent, explanatory variables only. In contrast, a plot of residuals identifies unusual observations in terms of the Y values we wish to explain.

> The hat matrix diagonal identifies leverage points with unusual values of the explanatory variables.

There are other high-leverage observations in the low-birth-weight baby data not apparent in Fig. 5.3. These observations appear near the center of this figure and are unusual in terms of explanatory variables other than length. Exercise 5.3 asks you to identify and explain these.

As an example of the hat matrix in practice, let us look at the code in Table 5.1 for the January temperature data. We can fit a linear model, plot the hat diagonals, and identify four most influential cities with this code

```
reg <- lm(JanTemp ~ Lat + Long + Alt, data = Jan)
inf <- influence(reg)
plot(reg$fitted.values, inf$hat, xlab = "Fitted values",
     ylab = "Hat diagonals")
ext <- match(sort(inf$hat)[leng - (0:3)], inf$hat)
text(reg$fitted.values[ext], inf$hat[ext],
     labels = row.names(Jan)[ext], pos = c(2, 4, 4, 2))
```

producing Fig. 5.4. The `influence` program takes the `lm` output and produces a number of diagnostic measures explained here. Other diagnostic measures are introduced in the following section.

Figure 5.4 plots the hat matrix diagonal against the fitted values (`reg$fitted .values`) for this regression model. This plot has the familiar U shape common to most hat matrix plots. We can intuit the extreme highest and lowest observed values of the explanatory variables are also furthest from the center of the data and will exert the greatest influence. Observations near the center of the data should generally have the least leverage.

When there are many explanatory variables, it is difficult to determine which observations are near the center and which are on the periphery. Identifying extreme points is especially difficult when this is the result of several of their explanatory variables, none of which is individually extreme. This is where the hat matrix and regression diagnostics described in the following section become most useful.

In the present plot for the January temperature data, Juneau and Honolulu have the most extreme longitude and latitude values and also have the highest leverage.

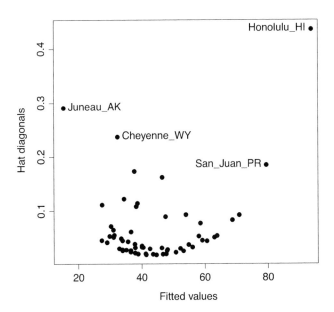

Figure 5.4 Hat matrix diagonal and fitted values for the January temperature data.

San Juan is far to the south of the continental United States and is also influential. Cheyenne is not the most extreme in terms of its fitted value, nor is it extreme in its latitude. However, many US cities are located at or near sea level, so the combined effects of extreme altitude and northern latitude of Cheyenne result in it exhibiting high leverage.

An informative graph in some situations is created by plotting the hat diagonals against the residuals of a model. The hat matrix identifies extremes in the explanatory variables and extreme residuals locate poorly fitted observations in terms of their response variable. Combining these two diagnostics allows us to identify poorly fitting observations and their leverage at the same time. The plot of residual and hat matrix diagonals for the January temperature data is given at the end of this chapter, in Fig. 5.8.

5.4   Jackknife Diagnostics

These are a set of useful diagnostic measures used to describe how influential an observation is on the overall fit of the model. The *jackknife* is a simple idea: delete an observation, refit the model without this observation, and then see how much the fitted model changes without it. This "leave one out" strategy is an intuitive idea to measure the influence of each observation. If an observation is deleted from the data set and the new fit is very different from the original model based on the full data set, then the omitted observation is said to be *influential* in the fit.

> The jackknife is a strategy to see how much the fitted model changes when each observation is deleted, in turn, and the model is refitted.

Each individual observation is deleted in turn, and then a new model is fitted corresponding to each deleted observation. The omitted observation is then replaced before the next observation is deleted. Many different things can change and a number of comparisons can be made between the model fitted with the full data and the model fitted from jackknifed data.

The `influence.measures` program produces several of the most popular diagnostics. Code for this appears in Output 5.3. The `influence.measures` program takes the output from the `lm` regression program to build a set of diagnostics. The `infmat` element is a matrix with a row for every observation in the original data and columns corresponding each of the various diagnostics.

Let's go over this list of the diagnostics produced by this **R** code. The last of these is the familiar hat matrix diagonal, covered in the previous section.

The `dffits` measures the change in the fitted value for each observation, both with and without this observation in the data. **R** will jackknife (delete) the ith observation, refit the model, and use these new fitted regression coefficients to estimate the value of the deleted observation. This jackknifed estimate is denoted by $\hat{y}_{(i)}$ where the

Output 5.3 Code to generate several useful regression diagnostics.

```
> reg <- lm(JanTemp ~ Lat + Long + Alt, data = Jan)
> im <- influence.measures(reg)$infmat
> im
                  dfb.1_ dfb.Lat dfb.Long  dfb.Alt   dffit  cov.r   cook.d   hat
Mobile_AL         0.0089 -0.0105  0.00111 -0.00403  0.0152  1.122 5.87e-05 0.0440
Montgomery_AL     0.0619 -0.0607 -0.00461 -0.02336  0.1027  1.085 2.67e-03 0.0326
Juneau_AK        -2.0655  1.5911  1.38848 -1.07121  2.2819  0.668 1.08e+00 0.2908
Pheonix_AZ       -0.0103 -0.1359  0.18911 -0.02720  0.2722  1.032 1.84e-02 0.0529
Little_Rock_AR   -0.0226  0.0299 -0.01277  0.02076 -0.0657  1.089 1.09e-03 0.0255
          ⋮                                            ⋮
                              ⋮
```

subscript in parentheses indicates the ith observation has been omitted. That is, $\hat{y}_{(i)}$ is the estimated value of y_i from the model fitted from data in which this observation has been deleted.

The `dffit` is equal to the difference

$$\hat{y}_i - \hat{y}_{(i)}$$

where the fitted observation $\hat{y}_i$ is estimated from the full data set. That is, the difference between the fitted value with, and then without, the specific observed value. This difference is standardized by the jackknifed hat matrix diagonal and mean square for residual in order to give the `dffit` a comparable variance for all observations.

A good strategy is to plot the `dffit` and look for any values with wide changes. Your visual inspection is probably the best way to judge problems with the data. As a rough rule of thumb, you should be suspicious of any observation with a `dffits` with an absolute value greater than

$$\sqrt{k/n},$$

where k is the number of parameters in the model and n is the sample size. Your own visual inspection should provide the best guidance.

The diagnostic called *Cook's D* combines all the individual `dffit` values for each observation into a single statistic. Cook's D measures how much all fitted values change when the ith observation is jackknifed.

Another useful jackknife diagnostic is the change in the estimated regression coefficients when an observation is deleted and the model is refitted. These are collectively called `dfbeta`. There will be a `dfbeta` for every observation and every regression parameter, including the intercept. When you run the program in Output 5.3 on your data, you will see the list of these variables and how **R** names these. The `dfbeta` changes in the estimated regression coefficients are standardized to make them comparable, but, as with the other diagnostics described in this section, your visual judgment is probably the best way to examine outliers among these values.

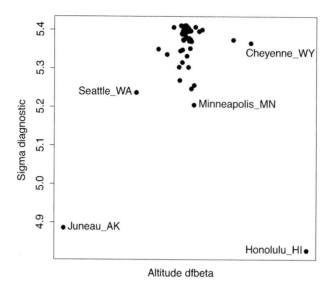

Figure 5.5 The `sigma` influence and altitude `dfbeta` for the January temperature data.

The covariance ratio is a jackknife measure of the stability of the estimated fitted values $\hat{Y}$. These are similar to the hat matrix diagonals discussed in Section 5.3 and are referred to as `cor.r` in **R**. Values of the covariance ratio should be close to 1 in value. These diagnostics are similar (but not identical) to the `dffit`.

One final diagnostic is the value of the standard deviation of the residuals when each observation is jackknifed. These values are obtained using code

```
reg <- lm(JanT ~ Lat + Long + Alt, data = Jan)   # fit original model
sig <- influence(reg)$sigma                       # sigma diagnostic
```

and the values are plotted in Fig. 5.5.

An influential observation usually also has high leverage, but a high leverage point does not have to be influential. In Fig. 4.3 (d), we see a set of high-leverage points, but deleting any one of these might not appreciably alter the fitted model. This is a subtle distinction, but in any case we should be prepared to identify unusual observations and explain why they are influential, have high leverage, or are outliers.

So, how do we make use of these different diagnostics? The short answer is some trial and error is necessary. Not all of these diagnostics will help identify unusual observations in every setting. One useful strategy is to plot one against another and use the resulting figure to identify influential observations in two directions at a time. An example of this is the plot of `sigma` influence and altitude `dfbeta` for the temperature data, given in Fig. 5.5.

In this figure we clearly see the cities Juneau and Honolulu, two very influential observations already identified. Other unusual cities appear to have influence and are identified. These include Cheyenne, a city with both very high altitude and latitude.

Also appearing in this figure is Seattle, a far northern city that is unusually warm (and rainy) due to Pacific currents.

More generally, what is a good way to proceed if we want to see what is happening in our data? First off, there is no one single rule to identify remarkable data points. All these methods rely on plotting the various diagnostics and using our vision to look for unusual patterns.

As for strategy, always begin by plotting your residuals. The residuals identify any major model failure including outliers failing to follow the overall pattern. Figure 4.3 is a good illustration of this.

A good second step is to examine the hat diagonal in order to identify leverage, or extremes, among the explanatory values. If the hat diagonal points out unusual observations, the jackknife diagnostics, especially the `dfbeta`, may be needed to identify how these influential observations came to your attention. Ultimately it remains up to you to explain the source of any unusual observations and how these data points should be treated.

5.5   Partial Correlation

In multiple linear regression there are several explanatory variables, and these will usually be correlated with each other. This leads us to ask how to attribute the contribution of each one toward explaining the outcome variable. In the low-birth-weight infant data, for example, length is useful in explaining birth weight. But length and birth weight are also related to the other variables in the data. There are a number of interesting relationships apparent in Fig. 2.13 between all the variables in the data set. How can we separate the contributions made by each of these individual explanatory variables?

At this point, we do not have a tool to address this question. The analysis of variance, for example, provides an F-ratio testing the null hypothesis that all population regression coefficients are equal to zero. This is useful in making a statement about the utility of the whole model, but it does not examine individual contributions. We can make use of regression output, as in Output 5.1, testing for statistical significance of individual regression coefficients, but this also fails to take into account the multivariate relationships between the various explanatory variables.

Let us start with the graphical display of the matrix scatter plot in Fig. 2.13. There's a lot going on, and we need a method to simplify things. We can start by computing all pairwise correlations given in Output 5.4, but this mass of numbers is not much clearer than the plots in Fig. 2.13.

A good way to display this correlation matrix is through the `corrplot` given in Fig. 5.6. The sizes of the dots are proportional to the magnitudes of the correlations. This figure was drawn in **R** using `corrplot(cor(baby))`. The `corrplot` function is very flexible and has many options you can read about in its `help` file. The `corrplot` function is in the **R** package of the same name and will have to be installed before using it it for the first time with `install.packages`.

Output 5.4 Correlations and partial correlations for low-birth-weight babies.

```
> cor(baby)                    #  correlation matrix
            head length   gage     wt momage pre.ecl
head      1.0000 0.7127 0.7807 0.7988 0.1321  0.1320
length    0.7127 1.0000 0.6752 0.8156 0.2180  0.1090
gage      0.7807 0.6752 1.0000 0.6599 0.2658  0.4120
wt        0.7988 0.8156 0.6599 1.0000 0.1546  0.0118
momage    0.1321 0.2180 0.2658 0.1546 1.0000  0.1141
pre.ecl   0.1320 0.1090 0.4120 0.0118 0.1141  1.0000
>
> pcor(baby)$estimate              #  partial correlations
            head  length   gage      wt  momage   pre.ecl
head      1.0000 0.01305 0.5447  0.4436 -0.1382 -0.14253
length    0.0131 1.00000 0.2007  0.5694  0.0994  0.00524
gage      0.5447 0.20068 1.0000  0.0358  0.2075  0.50258
wt        0.4436 0.56939 0.0358  1.0000 -0.0145 -0.19714
momage   -0.1382 0.09944 0.2075 -0.0145  1.0000 -0.02604
pre.ecl  -0.1425 0.00524 0.5026 -0.1971 -0.0260  1.00000
```

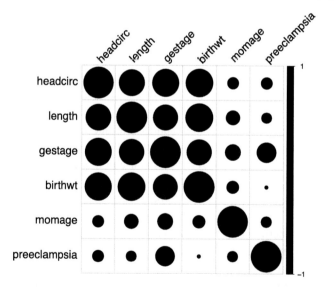

Figure 5.6 `corrplot` for low-birth-weight infants.

The largest dots in Fig. 5.6 are on the diagonal, corresponding to correlations of unity. The corrplot function reorders the variables to help identifying the group of measures (head circumference, length, gestational age, birth weight) which are all highly correlated. The other two measures (mother's age, pre-eclampsia) seem completely unrelated to either each other or any of the other variables in the data set.

If we have a number of intercorrelated variables, as in these data, we need a way to assess the individual contributions of one pair of measurements. As an example, there is a strong correlation (0.71) between head circumference and length, but these measures are also correlated with several other measures. So how much of this correlation is due to the confounding effects of the other values in the data?

We first need to remove the effects of all other variables on these two. Removing the effects means performing a linear regression on all other variables and then finding the correlation of their residuals. Formally, this procedure is called *partial correlation*.

Let's work out an example, again using the low-birth-weight infant data. For the partial correlation between length and head circumference, we first regress both of these variables on all others in the data set (but not each other), and then calculate the correlation of the residuals of the two regressions. That is, the partial correlation of length and head size is measured after we take into account the effects of all other variables in the data.

The partial correlation matrix is obtained in **R** by writing

```
pcor(baby)$estimate
```

using the pcor function in the ppcor library. These values appear in Output 5.4. The corrplot of these values is given in Fig. 5.7.

When we look at Fig. 5.7, we see the association between length and head circumference is quite small. The value of the partial correlation in Output 5.4 is almost zero (0.013), indicating the strong influence of the confounding variables in the data.

So, in summary, we see there is a high marginal correlation between the baby's length and head circumference. The marginal association refers to these two

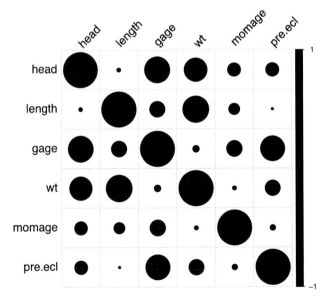

Figure 5.7 Partial correlation corrplot for low-birth-weight infants.

measurements taken by themselves. But as we have seen, almost all this association can be explained by the presence of other measurements in the data. The other measurements, in this case, are said to be confounded with the relationship. After removing the effects of the other variables, there is almost nothing left.

So, what exactly is the correlation between length and weight? The lesson from this exercise is to illustrate how it depends on the way this question is posed. The marginal correlation is very large but, at the same time, the partial correlation is almost zero. The length and weight measurements do not exist by themselves. In multiple linear regression, we need to think of individual observations as a multivariate object where all variables exhibit mutual interactions. A good analysis of the data discovers all of these relationships.

5.6   Model-Building Strategies

So far in this chapter we have learned how to use **R** and fit regressions with several explanatory variables. Sections 5.3 and 5.4 describe how to identify outliers and influential observations. In this section we describe the model-building process. When faced with many possible explanatory variables, how do we find a simple model explaining the dependent variable well? Which explanatory variables need to be included in the model? Which of these are not useful or are redundant?

There are several approaches we can take to make this task easier. The three we describe are stepwise selection (sometimes called *forward selection*), backward selection, and all possible regressions. In forward selection, the program adds explanatory variables to the model, one at a time, assessing their fit at each step. This proceeds until no variable not already in the model can be added to make a significant improvement.

In *backward selection*, the program begins with all possible explanatory variables in the model and then removes those not making a worthwhile contribution according to a specified criteria. In *all possible regressions,* as the name implies, the program fits all possible models and then presents several among the best of these.

Let us illustrate stepwise regression using the low-birth-weight data. Recall we are building a model to be used to explain the different birth weights of the infants in this data set. The program lines

```
fit <- lm(wt ~ head + length + gage + momage + pre.ecl, data = baby)
ols_step_forward_p(fit)
```

requests **R** to perform a forward selection procedure.

A portion of the output from this program is given in Output 5.5. At the first step, the infant length variable was included in the model. At the next two steps, the head circumference and then the indication of pre-eclampsia were added. No further variables were found to make a statistical contribution, and the model building stopped at that point. At each successive step we see the R^2 increases but the final addition of pre-eclampsia only provides a small improvement. Similar statements can be made about the other measures of fit as well.

Output 5.5 A portion of the forward stepwise regression output for the low-birth-weight baby data.

```
                          Selection Summary
------------------------------------------------------------------
         Variable              Adj.
Step     Entered    R-Square  R-Square   C(p)       AIC        RMSE
------------------------------------------------------------------
  1      length      0.6651    0.6617   42.0945   1299.0624   157.0359
  2      head        0.7613    0.7564    4.4209   1267.1938   133.2544
  3      pre.ecl     0.7717    0.7646    2.1258   1264.7317   130.9913
------------------------------------------------------------------
```

The stepwise model-building process ends at the point when length, head circumference, and pre-eclampsia are in the model. The omitted variables (gestational age and mother's age) are judged to have no additional explanatory value, given the other three variables already in the linear model.

The `ols_step_forward_p` program and all the stepwise programs in this section are in the `olsrr` package which must be installed before use. Each of these programs produces more output than given in Output 5.5. There are also options to plot the summary statistics at each step to allow us to judge the progress of the stepwise process.

Backward stepwise regression is similar to forward stepwise, except it begins with all possible explanatory variables in the model and then removes, one at a time, those making the least contribution. The **R** code for running a backward regression is as follows.

```
ols_step_backward_p(fit)
```

We will not include the output from this program, but it ends at the same place as the forward selection method: first removing the mother's age and then removing gestational age from the model.

Some fans of stepwise regression prefer the backward method over forward selection because every explanatory variable gets a chance of being included in the final model. Others might argue backward regression is unnecessarily complicated right at the beginning. In this example of the low-birth-weight infants, both the forward and backward programs end at the same place, namely the model with same three explanatory variables: length, head circumference, and pre-eclampsia. In this example it doesn't matter which stepwise direction was used, because both come to the same conclusion. This might not be the case in other examples.

In further refinements of forward stepwise regression, some strategies may allow for the exclusion of a variable once it is included. Similarly, backward stepwise regression might later consider including a variable again after it has been removed.

Critics of stepwise methods will be quick to remind you the level of statistical significance will be distorted because a number of significance tests have been performed without taking their multiplicity into account. A discussion of multiplicity of tests and their Bonferroni correction is given in Section 2.4. Even if we were willing to make this correction, it is not clear how many comparisons were made by the stepwise procedure.

It is possible neither forward nor backward methods obtain the best model. We might also wonder how far the best is from second best or whether a much simpler model might do almost as well. This is the approach taken by the all-possible-regressions method. Before we explain the all-possible-regressions method, let us explain some criteria we might use to decide what we mean by *best*.

In the present section, there are a number of statistics cited in order to gauge how well our model fits. The fact there are different methods suggests these methods are not always in agreement, and the criteria used to judge quality are often subjective. The general agreement, however, is simplicity wins.

> There is a penalty for building overly complicated models.

A model with many explanatory variables will confuse your audience. A model with almost as many estimated parameters as observations will fit the data well but does not simplify things. Complicated rules do not produce a better summary of the data.

Fitting a model with a large number of explanatory variables can result in an unrealistically large R^2 statistic. Adding a large number of explanatory variables can inflate this statistic. In model building, it is not fair to compare two models with different numbers of explanatory variables, because the larger model will have an unfair advantage. It seems intuitive a price should be paid for providing an unnecessarily complex model with the purpose of simplifying the data. At the extreme, if each observation is used to explain its own value, then the R^2 will equal 1. Such a model is useless. See Exercise 5.1 for more information about such a strategy for model building.

The *adjusted* R^2 statistic takes the number of explanatory variables p into account. The definition is

$$\text{Adjusted } (R^2) = 1 - \frac{(N-1)(1-R^2)}{N-p},$$

where R^2 is the usual or unadjusted value, p is the number of parameters in the model, and N is the sample size.

If the sample size N is much larger than the number of explanatory variables, then the adjusted R^2 will not be very different from the usual R^2. **R** prints out both the R^2 and the adjusted R^2 in the output from most programs. If these two statistics are very different in value, then this indicates an overly fitted model with too many explanatory variables, relative to the sample size.

Another useful statistic in model building is C_p, defined as

$$C_p = \frac{\text{Error SS}(p \text{ parameter model})}{s^2(\text{for the full model})} - N + 2p,$$

where s^2 is the mean square for error of the full model and N and p are the sample size and number of explanatory variables, as before. Values of C_p are given in Output 5.5.

This statistic is used to compare a full model including all the explanatory variables to a smaller model with p parameters. Smaller values of C_p are preferred, because these represent both a small root-mean-square error of the model and fewer terms in the model.

There are a large number of other criteria to judge models and compare one with another. These are beyond our present needs and so we will return to model building in **R**.

In addition to stepwise regression, *all possible regressions* is another popular automated model-building strategy. In all possible regressions, we can fit every possible regression model by alternately including and excluding every combination of the explanatory variables listed in the `model` statement. To obtain the all-possible-regressions model in **R**, we write

```
ols_step_all_possible(fit)
```

and we can identify the best of these using the following.

```
ols_step_best_subset(fit)
```

Let us conclude this section with a brief discussion of the methods covered here. In each of the three methods (forward, backward, and all possible) described in this section for building a regression model, we are asking the computer to decide which variables to include in our model. The automation of the process is both easy to do and intuitive.

This also relieves us of some of the responsibility we have for our data. We often have some good knowledge of the variables involved and their relationships with each other and the dependent variable. Why was data on each of the variables collected? Was there a reason for each variable's inclusion in the data set, or did somebody suggest we collect as much as we could in the hope something might prove to be useful?

In the field of *data mining*, researchers start with huge databases and look for any and all useful patterns. With many possible choices for models, it is easy to find a statistically significant model. However, we also need to make sure the model makes practical sense, or it will not provide any useful value.

> We are not finished with any regression until we
> interpret our final model.

We cannot simply say a model is the one the computer suggested. Besides the diagnostics (outliers, residuals, influence) discussed earlier in this chapter, we also need to be able to defend the model in terms of the underlying science of the problem giving rise to the data. Does the model make sense? Do the explanatory variables in the model have some valid or intuitive reason for being there? As pointed out in Section 4.5.4, statistics is more than numbers.

5.7   Exercises

5.1   Consider a model with just as many explanatory variables as observations. How many degrees of freedom would the residual sums of squares have? What would be the numerical value of the residual sums of squares in this setting? What would the value of the unadjusted R^2 be? Similarly, how can we make the R^2 large? Is this a useful strategy for building a model of our data?

5.2   Look at the arsenic exposure data in Exercise 3.5.2 and examine whether there are differences in sexes. Is the self-reported amount of well water used for drinking and cooking useful in explaining toenail arsenic levels? In Exercise 4.5 we identified an influential observation in these data with an extremely high exposure level. Do your conclusions change when this person is deleted from the regression model? Should this person's data be deleted in order to meet the assumptions of the statistical model? Do the jackknife diagnostics tell you anything else? Is it possible this observation is the most important and informative of all?

5.3   Examine the low-birth-weight infant data using all the explanatory variables available. Plot the hat matrix diagonal against the fitted value and notice two very influential observations. One of these influential observations had an extreme length and is identified in Fig. 5.3. Locate one other observation with an extremely large influence. Notice this second infant is neither extreme in length nor in weight. Why is this observation influential?

5.4   Reexamine the baseball attendance figures in Table 3.1. Does the size of payroll influence the finishing position? Does the finishing position of the team affect the average attendance? Does pay result in performance? Does performance result in increased attendance? What happens if we include the effects of market size, measured by population in the metropolitan area? Are there outlier teams or teams exhibiting influence in your regression?

5.7.1   University Endowments

Universities need plenty of money to operate. Not all of this is covered by tuition and grants. University endowments act as large savings accounts used as needed for building new and refurbishing existing facilities, and to hire new faculty and staff. Most

Table 5.2 The largest university endowments, 2017.

| Institution | Endowment in $ Billion | | | % change | 2015 student | Endowment per |
	2017	2016	2015	2016–17	body size	student in $M
Harvard	36.02	34.54	36.45	4.28	21,000	1.74
Yale	27.18	25.41	25.57	6.95	12,336	2.07
U Texas	26.54	24.20	24.08	9.64	216,000	0.11
Stanford	24.79	22.40	22.22	10.66	16,795	1.32
Princeton	23.81	22.15	22.72	7.49	8,088	2.81
MIT	14.97	13.18	13.48	13.55	11,319	1.19
U Pennsylvania	12.21	10.72	10.13	13.98	21,296	0.48
Texas A&M	11.56	10.54	10.48	9.64	143,000	0.07
U Michigan	10.94	9.74	9.95	12.24	43,625	0.23
Northwestern	10.44	9.65	10.19	8.18	20,336	0.50
Columbia	10.00	9.04	9.64	10.57	29,870	0.32
Notre Dame	9.35	8.37	8.57	11.68	12,179	0.70
U Virginia	8.62	5.85	6.18	47.32	23,732	0.26
Duke	7.91	6.84	7.30	15.66	14,850	0.49
Washington, U./ St. Louis	7.86	6.46	6.82	21.63	14,503	0.47
UChicago	7.52	7.00	7.55	7.47	15,244	0.50
Emory	6.91	6.40	6.68	7.86	14,769	0.45
Cornell	6.76	5.76	6.04	17.37	21,850	0.28

Source: National Association of College and University Business Officers, 2017.

of the money comes either as contributions from alumni or as returns on investments. Some of these endowments have grown to huge sizes over the years. Data on the 10 largest endowments (in 2017) is given in Table 5.2.

This table provides data on the largest total endowments along with their change over the previous year, and the share of the endowment on a per-student basis. We can obtain an approximation to the number of students in the university using the ratio

$$\text{Number of students} = 1000 \times \frac{\text{Endowment}}{\text{Endowment per student}}.$$

We multiply this ratio by 1000 because the endowments are measured in billions of dollars but the per-student values are in millions.

The amount of a university endowment is principally due to return on investments and, to a smaller degree, to contributions from former students and their families. Similarly, the percent change over the previous year's endowment is also made up of these two factors. Build a linear model and see if you can explain the 2017 endowment value from the number of current students and the percent change over the previous year.

Which of the explanatory variables offers greater value in explaining the size of the endowments? Similarly, does this data help explain whether universities put more effort into raising money from former students or seeking greater investment returns?

5.7.2   Maximum January Temperatures

Plot a map of the United States by drawing a scatter plot of the latitude and longitude values. Where are Miami, New York, Juneau, and Honolulu? Are they where they should be?

Fit a linear model explaining different temperatures from the other covariates. Plot your residuals and look for outliers. Explain these. Identify influential points using the diagnostics described in this chapter. Explain any influential observations you find.

What role does the intercept play? Does its value have meaning? Hint: Look at a world map to find the location with a zero latitude, longitude, and altitude. Learn why residents of Ghana claim to live near the center of the earth.

Try putting both longitude and longitude-squared in the same model. Try something nobody else thought of. Does your R-squared or root-mean-squared error improve your ability to explain the temperature values? What evidence can you provide your model is any good?

There are some very large outliers in this data. Carefully identify these cities. Large positive and negative residuals occur in Juneau and Honolulu. These observations are also highly influential, as we see in Fig. 5.8. Are you surprised to learn the identity of the outliers? Does your intuition help you or hinder you? Can you explain why these residuals are so extreme in their respective directions?

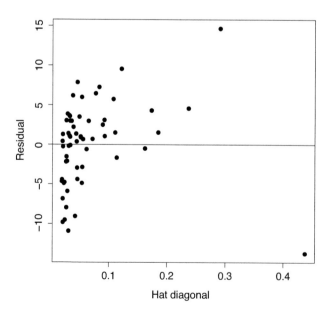

Figure 5.8 Hat matrix diagonal and residuals for the maximum January temperature data.

Table 5.3 Hospital costs and mortality following bypass surgery in a survey of hospitals in the Philadelphia area. Death rates are summarized as being greater than (+), lower than (−), or close to (0) expected.

Hospital	Average paid to hospital		Postsurgical length of stay (days)	Cases	In-hospital deaths	
	By Medicare	By private insurance			Number	Rate
Lower Bucks	30	95	7.1	74	2	0
Hahnemann University	50	78	8.1	153	9	+
Albert Einstein	45	73	6.1	116	6	+
Graduate	40	70	5.2	43	2	+
Crozer-Chester	35	66	5.8	102	1	0
U of Pa Hospital	45	62	6.6	145	3	0
Temple University	42	58	7.1	114	4	0
Thomas Jefferson Univ	43	50	7.6	173	3	0
Main Line Paoli	30	45	6.5	105	3	0
Penn Presbyterian	35	43	6.5	221	5	0
Mercy Fitzgerald	42	45	7.0	90	9	+
Brandywine	30	43	5.3	57	1	0
Pennsylvania	39	41	6.5	91	5	0
Abington Memorial	37	37	7.2	153	6	0
Main Line Bryn Mawr	30	36	6.3	86	4	0
Main Line Lankenau	30	35	5.4	299	2	−
Frankford	38	30	6.5	231	1	0
Doylestown	25	30	5.6	182	2	0
Chester County	29	24	5.8	91	1	0
Phoenixville	.	18	5.5	60	0	0

Source: Pennsylvania Health Care Cost Containment Council.

5.7.3   Heart Surgery Mortality

Table 5.3 presents a summary of survey data obtained from hospitals in the Philadelphia area in 2005. The newspaper article[1] concentrates on coronary bypass surgery and the costs of patient care. The article questions whether the mortality outcome is related to the cost of the procedure.

This table provides the following data variables.

- Average costs paid by Medicare.
- Average costs paid by private insurance.
- Average postsurgical length of hospital stay, in days.
- Number of cases treated.
- Number of in-hospital deaths.

---

[1] Available online at www.nytimes.com/2007/06/14/health/14insure.html.

The number of deaths should always be expressed as a rate, or the ratio of the number of deaths to the number of cases. Otherwise, hospitals treating the most patients would also appear to have the most deaths.

Consider the average total cost per patient as your dependent variable. Total cost is the sum of the amounts paid by Medicare and private insurance. Is the average number of hospital days related to the average total costs paid by insurers? Suppose you use the average length of hospital stay as your dependent variable. Can this variable be explained well by the average costs paid?

Create a new variable as the ratio of Medicare to private insurance costs for each hospital. Is this ratio related to either length of stay or mortality rate? Private insurance patients are more likely to be employed or have greater financial means. Hospitals with greater private insurance claims may also have healthier patients than hospitals with a larger percentage of Medicare reimbursements.

This table also includes a column indicating whether the mortality was higher or lower than expected. Do you agree with these measures? Do these summaries correspond to the residuals in your regression model? Another examination of the mortality data in this figure is given in Section 10.6.1.

5.7.4   Characteristics of Cars, 1974

Let's go back to the days when leaded gasoline cost less than $1.00, before catalytic converters, back to the time of an earlier energy crisis, back when Nissan was called Datsun. But look: after all these years, Toyota still makes the Corolla.

The data in Table 5.4 lists 10 different characteristics of cars manufactured in 1973–4. The data was originally published in a 1974 issue of *Motor Trend* magazine, and other statistical analysis have appeared. Besides the make and model, these are the variables:

- mpg: miles per US gallon
- cyl: number of cylinders
- disp: displacement (in cubic inches)
- hp: gross horsepower

Table 5.4 Characteristics of cars in 1974.

Make and Model	mpg	cyl	disp	hp	rar	wt	qsec	V/S	T	G	C
Mazda RX4	21.0	6	160.0	110	3.90	2.620	16.46	0	1	4	4
Mazda RX4 Wag	21.0	6	160.0	110	3.90	2.875	17.02	0	1	4	4
Datsun 710	22.8	4	108.0	93	3.85	2.320	18.61	1	1	4	1
Toyota Corolla	33.9	4	71.1	65	4.22	1.835	19.90	1	1	4	1
⋮											
Volvo 142E	21.4	4	121.0	109	4.11	2.780	18.60	1		1	4	2

Source: mtcars in the **R data sets** library.

- rar: rear axle ratio
- wt: weight (lb/1000)
- qsec: 1/4 mile time
- V/S: cylinders form a "V" (= 1) or are in a straight line (= 0)
- T: transmission (0 = automatic, 1 = manual)
- G: number of forward gears
- C: number of carburetors.

Much can be said about the data, and a variety of analyses are possible. Much will be left to the reader's creativity, and a few simple plots will reveal many details. Here are a few suggestions to get you started.

- Begin with a matrix scatter plot (as in Fig. 5.1) to reveal any obvious strong pairwise relationships.
- The quarter mile times have outliers at both the high and low ends. What are the characteristics of cars exhibiting these extremes?
- A plot of disp against rar reveals two distinct groups of cars. How can these be distinguished?
- A plot of weight and displacement reveals either three very influential observations, or possibly three distinct groups of cars.
- Miles per gallon is negatively correlated with horsepower, but note there are a few exceptions to the overall pattern.

Don't aim for a complete and thorough analysis of these data – that could take a very long time. It is better to concentrate on some aspect and provide a clear story conveying both your understanding of the data and the statistical methods employed.

5.7.5   Statistics in Advertising: Wine Prices

For those of us whose expertise in wine consists of telling reds from whites, there are experts who rate wines and give them a score. Higher scores are better, and 99 or 100 is the maximum. Naturally, merchants will advertise high scores in an attempt to charge higher prices.

Table 5.5 shows a list of wines from an advertisement appearing in the *New York Times*, May 1, 2005. The prices in Table 5.5 are per bottle. It would seem the ad appeals to consumers who would seek a rating of 90 or higher. That is, the advertisement ends at this value. Such data is called *censored* because certain values are not observed. Recall the low-birth-weight data of Section 3.1 is also censored. We discuss censored data again when we describe the analysis of survival data in Chapter 11.

Three columns are in Table 5.5: points, year of vintage, and price. In every case, the sale price is one cent less than the value listed here, so the first item sells for $599.99 instead of the $600 listed here. The one bottle with a $1400 price is not an error.

The vintage years omit the century number. Output 5.6 provides a program to read the data correctly and fix the year number.

Table 5.5 Rating points, vintage year and price for bottles of wine in an advertisement.

Pts	Year	Price	Pts	Year	Price	Pts	Year	Price	Pts	Year	Price
99	00	600	99	96	500	99	89	350	99	86	625
99	00	600	99	90	500	99	90	500	99	00	550
99	91	250	99	01	190	99	83	550	99	90	400
99	96	450	99	95	150	99	82	500	98	86	450
98	98	250	98	02	200	98	03	350	98	00	80
98	01	70	97	98	200	97	01	90	97	00	190
97	00	300	97	02	275	96	03	100	96	00	330
96	01	80	96	01	100	96	00	300	96	02	40
95	01	70	95	01	150	95	97	550	95	97	100
95	01	100	95	01	225	95	01	550	95	97	90
95	01	130	95	01	70	95	00	120	95	00	180
95	98	260	95	01	100	95	01	140	95	02	45
95	03	80	95	99	85	95	03	100	95	97	100
95	99	70	95	99	70	95	01	150	95	00	230
95	98	100	94	01	140	94	96	60	94	99	70
94	98	190	94	01	100	94	01	80	94	02	70
94	03	70	94	00	60	94	01	60	94	01	120
94	99	80	94	99	90	94	01	140	94	99	500
94	99	70	94	99	80	94	01	130	94	01	140
94	86	200	94	99	200	94	01	240	94	00	140
94	01	80	93	02	125	93	02	270	93	02	540
93	01	600	93	99	80	93	98	80	93	98	50
93	99	1400	93	98	125	93	01	130	93	00	55
93	89	150	93	00	140	93	03	30	93	02	100
93	99	60	93	99	130	93	01	50	93	00	40
93	99	50	93	01	75	93	01	240	93	01	100
93	00	30	92	02	65	92	00	50	92	01	35
92	01	60	92	02	40	92	99	90	92	02	27
92	00	400	92	00	70	92	00	120	92	00	60
92	01	75	92	02	53	92	00	70	92	98	70
92	02	80	92	98	60	92	99	50	92	99	60
92	00	100	92	99	60	92	99	50	92	00	70
92	98	60	92	02	28	92	02	22	92	01	35
92	02	70	92	96	60	92	00	70	92	00	48
92	02	28	91	01	35	91	03	30	91	99	80
91	01	25	91	99	50	91	01	35	91	02	18
91	01	50	91	03	16	91	01	30	91	01	27
91	01	130	91	00	75	91	03	19	91	00	275
91	02	37	91	02	50	91	02	50	91	02	35
91	00	19	91	03	40	91	03	27	91	02	60
91	02	40	91	02	50	91	02	35	91	02	20
91	02	40	91	02	50	90	01	10	90	03	13
90	01	18	90	02	13	90	01	40	90	01	20
90	02	17	90	01	24	90	02	19	90	03	13
90	01	40	90	01	45	90	01	19	90	02	18
90	02	20	90	02	30						

Output 5.6 R code to read wine price data.

```
> wine <- scan(file = "wine.dat")     #  read data as a list
Read 546 items
> n <- length(wine)/3                  #  number of items in the list
> wine <- t(matrix(wine, c(3, n)))     #  express as nx3 matrix
> wine <- data.frame(wine)
> colnames(wine) <- c("rating", "year", "price")
> wine[1:10, ]                              # first ten rows
     rating year price
1       99    0   600
2       99   96   500
3       99   89   350
4       99   86   625
5       99    0   600
6       99   90   500
7       99   90   500
8       99    0   550
9       99   91   250
10      99    1   190
> wine$year <- wine$year + 1900 + 100 * (wine$year < 20) # correct year
> wine[1:10, ]                              # ten rows with correct year
     rating year price
1       99 2000   600
2       99 1996   500
3       99 1989   350
4       99 1986   625
5       99 2000   600
6       99 1990   500
7       99 1990   500
8       99 2000   550
9       99 1991   250
10      99 2001   190
```

Perform a linear regression using only year and point score to explain the price. Look at the regression coefficients and interpret these. How much of a price difference is one year worth? Explain why one of these regression coefficients is positive and the other is negative.

Which is more important in determining price: older vintage or better rating? What is the trade-off in price for age and rating: how many years is one point worth? Is the point scale linear in price, or does there appear to be a larger price difference as the points become larger? For example, is the difference in price between 90 and 92 the same as the difference between 96 and 98? Does every year have the same distribution of high and low ranks or were some years better than others? Can you identify bargains and/or overpriced wines?

Look at the residuals for this model and plot the residuals against the fitted value. Notice how the $1400 wine distorts the figure. Delete this wine and run the regression again. How does the R^2 change? Can you explain this? Does the root mean square change when you delete the most expensive wine? How do you interpret this? Examine the measures of influence and identify any other unusual observations. Did you notice there is a wine with a negative estimated price? How do you explain this? *Cheers!*

5.7.6   Statistics in Finance: Mutual Fund Returns

Mutual funds are a convenient way for many investors to pool their savings and participate in the stock market. A fund manager invests the money and keeps records. For this work, the manager is paid an annual fee out of the funds being managed. This fee is called the *expense ratio* and is usually a fraction of 1%. The records (at the time of this writing) of the largest mutual funds investing in large corporations are given in Table 5.6.

Table 5.6 The 25 largest mutual funds investing in the stocks of large corporations. The types are Growth, Value, and Blend.

Name	Type	% Total annual return 1 year	% Total annual return 5 years	Expense ratio	Assets ($ million)
Amer Funds Growth Fund A	G	14.4	15.6	0.63	94,406
Fidelity Contrafund	G	20.8	17.7	0.89	82,646
Amer Funds Inv Co	V	8.5	13.1	0.54	78,309
Amer Funds Washington	V	6.6	12.4	0.57	71,169
Dodge & Cox Stock	V	2.9	16.2	0.52	68,711
Vanguard 500 Index	B	7.4	12.3	0.18	68,416
Vanguard Total Stock	B	7.6	13.6	0.19	50,929
Vanguard Inst Indx	B	7.5	12.4	0.05	47,686
Fidelity Magellan	G	20.4	11.9	0.53	47,337
Fidelity Growth Company	G	23.3	18.4	0.96	39,106
Amer Funds Fundamental	B	14.9	18.1	0.58	38,851
Vanguard Windsor II	V	6.4	15.2	0.33	33,821
Fidelity Equity Income	V	4.2	13.5	0.67	32,540
Davis NY Venture A	B	6.4	14.8	0.84	32,138
Fidelity Spar US Eq Inv	B	7.5	12.3	0.09	24,106
Vanguard PRIMECAP	G	13.5	17.0	0.46	23,989
T. Rowe Price Gr Stk	G	12.5	13.6	0.70	22,136
T. Rowe Price Eq Inc	V	5.0	13.5	0.69	21,977
Fidelity Growth & Income	B	3.1	8.1	0.67	21,794
Fidelity Blue Chip	G	13.9	9.6	0.59	18,940
Amer Funds Amcap A	G	10.5	12.2	0.65	18,913
Amer Funds Amer Mut A	V	6.0	12.1	0.55	17,747
Lord Abbott Affiliated A	V	6.2	13.4	0.82	16,802
Fidelity Dividend Growth	B	4.6	9.2	0.60	16,387
Vanguard Windsor	V	1.9	14.4	0.35	14,489

Source: New York Times, November 6, 2007, page C10.

The two basic approaches to investing in stocks are *growth* and *value*. Growth stocks are in companies with the potential for new discoveries or products leading to large increases in their future income. Value stocks represent bargains in which the price does not fully reflect the true worth of the share of the underlying corporation. In some years one approach may be a much better investment than the other, but over time there is generally little difference in the returns. In the one year leading up to the data in this table, growth stocks performed much better, but in the few years before that, value stocks did better. Blended funds invest in both of these types. Some of the mutual funds in this table emphasize current income, and others look for potential gains at some future date.

What determines the total assets of the fund? We can think of the total assets as a collection of many decisions made by the investors, who could easily move their money elsewhere if they became dissatisfied with the service the manager is providing. Which is more important in determining the total assets of a fund: the expense ratio or the return the fund has experienced? That is, are investors more interested in the history of the fund or the amount they will have to pay for performance? Similarly, are larger expenses associated with better returns?

Consider other relationships in this data. Do value managers provide lower expense ratios? We might ask if value managers themselves provide value to their investors. Is the one-year return correlated with the five-year return? Why would you expect this to be the case? Is this correlation the same for value and growth managers? Can you identify funds performing well under all conditions, regardless of whether growth or value stocks provide the best returns?

6 Indicators, Interactions, and Transformations

Linear regression is sometimes more than we really need. A simple rule of thumb is often adequate. When you look at the fuel gauge on your car, at what point do you begin to look for a gas station? Which is more useful: the gauge or the warning light? An indicator variable takes a continuous measurement and cuts it up into two discrete categories.

We can also transform variables in a nonlinear fashion if this serves to reduce leverage or make the data look more like a straight line. Interactions are variables we use in a regression model to see if the explanatory value of two variables is greater than the sum of their parts. A pizza with two toppings may be much better than two separate halves with the individual toppings. Or perhaps it may be worse.

6.1   Indicator Variables

Water boils at a lower temperature at high altitude, and experienced cooks know recipes need to be adjusted accordingly. Consider the recipe given in Table 6.1. Most important, notice the footnote about making an adjustment for high altitude. This is expressed in terms of a change needing to be made above a critical height above sea level. Ideally, the person preparing this dish should first obtain an accurate measure of the barometric pressure and then calculate the precise amount of adjustment to be made. Nobody would consider doing this, of course. Instead we are instructed to use this easily remembered rule taking effect above a critical level.

Let us take the January temperature data described in Chapter 5 and see how to create and interpret an indicator variable. The estimated regression coefficients in Table 5.1 show average temperature drops about two degrees Fahrenheit for every degree latitude North a city is located. Suppose we want to create a simple rule about the temperature in northern and southern cities, much like the one in the recipe. That is, what simple statement can we make about northern and southern cities not involving a calculation?

We can pick any cut point we want, so let us choose Washington, DC, at 38 degrees latitude as the division between northern and southern cities. This choice is intuitive,

Table 6.1 Recipe for Hamburger Helper Lasagna.

YOU WILL NEED:
1 lb lean ground beef
3 1/4 cups hot water
1. BROWN ground beef in 10-inch skillet; drain.
2. STIR in hot water, Sauce Mix and uncooked Pasta.
    HEAT to boiling; stirring occasionally.
3. REDUCE heat; cover and simmer about 14 minutes,
    stirring occasionally, until pasta is tender.
    REMOVE from heat and uncover (sauce will thicken as it stands).

HIGH ALTITUDE (3500–6500 ft) Increase hot water to 3 1/2 cups and
simmer time to about 15 min.

Copyright General Foods Corporation, used with permission.

but it is also arbitrary. We could just as well pick a different division. Notice we are picking the place to make the cut, and the computer is not estimating it for us. The **R** program to create the new variable and perform regression using it is given in Output 6.1.

A regression analysis of these data also appears in Output 5.1. The data is read in this program into a `dataframe` called `city`. The **R** code here creates a new variable called DC taking values TRUE and FALSE, depending on whether the latitude is greater than or less than 38. The program prints the first five of these to show this is the case. It is always good practice to check the coding was done correctly.

We can can also convert DC to 0/1 values. Several ways to do this are to multiply the logical values in DC by 1; add 0 to DC; or use the function `as.numeric(DC)` In any case, we can regress on the DC variable, expressed as either logical or numeric.

Such a variable is called an *indicator* or *dummy*, because it is not a real observed value, but rather an artificial one we constructed. It operates much like a light switch, with only two positions. The DC variable is created using a logical operation. The statement `city$Lat > 38` is either true or false for each of the cities.

After creating the new indicator called DC, we are free to use it as we would use any other variable in a linear regression. For simplicity, this is the only explanatory variable in the present regression model. Output 6.1 contains the **R** code and output with the estimated regression coefficients for this model.

How do we interpret the fitted model and estimated regression coefficients? The estimated intercept is about 57 and the slope is -23, but what does this mean? If we write out the model, then it will become clear.

The fitted regression equation is

$$\text{maximum January temperature} = 57 - 23 \times \text{DC}.$$

Output 6.1 **R** program to create and regress on an indicator variable for latitude north of Washington, DC (38 degrees, latitude).

```
> city <- read.table(file = "Jan.txt", header = T, row.names = 5)
> city[1:5, ]                        # echo the first few
                JanT Lat Long  Alt
Mobile_AL         61  30   88    5
Montgomery_AL     59  32   86  160
Juneau_AK         30  58  134   50
Pheonix_AZ        64  33  112 1090
Little_Rock_AR    51  34   92  286
> DC <- (city$Lat > 38)              # indicate north of DC
> DC[1:5]                            # verify the first of these
[1] FALSE FALSE  TRUE FALSE FALSE
>
> reg <- lm(JanT ~ DC, data = city) # regress on this indicator
> summary(reg)

Call:
lm(formula = JanT ~ DC, data = city)

Residuals:
    Min     1Q  Median     3Q     Max
-17.077  -6.077  -1.029  5.971  23.923

Coefficients:
              Estimate Std. Error t value Pr(>|t|)
(Intercept)     57.077      1.784  31.985  < 2e-16 ***
DCTRUE         -23.048      2.356  -9.784  5.8e-14 ***
---
Signif. codes:  0 '***' 0.001 '**' 0.01 '*' 0.05 '.' 0.1 ' ' 1

Residual standard error: 9.099 on 59 degrees of freedom
Multiple R-squared:  0.6187, Adjusted R-squared:  0.6122
F-statistic: 95.72 on 1 and 59 DF,  p-value: 5.799e-14
```

When DC $= 0$, or FALSE we have, on average,

$$\text{maximum January temperature} = 57$$

as the estimate for all cities south of Washington.

Similarly, when DC $= 1$, or TRUE, the regression model estimates

$$\text{maximum January temperature} = 57 - 23 = 34$$

is the average maximum January temperature for cities north of Washington.

Output 6.2 The regression in Output 6.1 performed as a t-test.

```
> t.test(city$JanT[DC], city$JanT[ !DC], var.equal = T)

Two Sample t-test

data:  city$JanT[DC] and city$JanT[!DC]
t = -9.7836, df = 59, p-value = 5.799e-14
alternative hypothesis: true difference in means is not equal to 0
95 percent confidence interval:
 -27.76234 -18.33436
sample estimates:
mean of x mean of y
 34.02857  57.07692
```

In words, the regression slope on the indicator variable DC is the difference of two means. We can verify the estimated slope is exactly the same as the difference of two means obtained in a Student t-test using the program of Output 6.2. This demonstrates the close connection between the t-test and the use of indicator variables in linear regression. The assumption of constant variance in regression is carried into the t-test using the var.equal = T option in Output 6.2.

We can use regression to perform a t-test, but the real benefit of indicator variables is the improved ease of interpretation, as we see in the difference between northern and southern cities as well as in the recipe in Table 6.1. In both examples, a continuous variable (latitude and altitude, respectively) has been cut into two categories, resulting in a simple, easy-to-explain rule.

How much is lost or gained by creating the indicator variable in this example? At the analytic level, we can show the residual sum of squares is larger for a regression model with the DC variable than if we regressed directly on latitude. This shows the model with latitude is more precise and has better explanatory value. There is a price to be paid for this benefit, however.

The first part of the price is the added difficulty we have with the final fitted model. Recall the ease we have with the simple rule about the altitude adjustment in the recipe. The second advantage of using an indicator variable in this example is the influence of extreme latitude values is eliminated. If we look back at Fig. 5.8, we see the cities at extreme latitudes (Juneau and Honolulu) are also the most influential by using the hat matrix diagonal. The use of an indicator variable with only two values will eliminate the influence of extreme latitude values. There are advantages and penalties to using either approach, and the user should recognize these.

Let us next create an indicator with more than two categories. Categorical explanatory variables appear often in data analysis. These may be obtained as the unordered categories of race or religion, for examples. The categories might also be ordered as in the previous example of latitude divided up into two or more ordered groups. The use of indicator variables can help interpret the data if performed carefully.

Let us examine the January temperature again and consider dividing the altitude variable into three categories. Many cities are located at or near sea level, so let us define a category for cities at 100 feet or less above sea level. Those in the Rocky Mountains tend to more than 1000 feet above sea level. The remaining cities are in the middle, neither at high altitude nor at sea level. These distinctions are somewhat arbitrary but lend themselves to ease of interpretation.

The **R** code to create the three binary-valued indicators is as follows.

```
sea <- (city$Alt <= 100)  +0
mid <- ((city$Alt >100) & (city$Alt <1000)) + 0
high <- (city$Alt >= 1000) +0
```

This code creates a variable called sea indicating a city at sea level, a variable called mid identifying cities located between 100 and 1000 feet, and a variable called high equal to 1 for cities above or equal to 1000 feet. The characters <= are interpreted as "less than or equal to." The ampersand & performs the logical AND operation. We add zero to each of these indicators to convert T/F values into numeric 1/0.

We can use these indicators in a regression model, but first let us point out a problem occurs if we try to use all three in the same model.

If we try to fit the model

$$\texttt{lm(JanT ~ sea + mid +high, data = city)}$$

in **R**, then the mathematical model

$$\texttt{JanT} = \alpha + \beta_1\texttt{sea} + \beta_2\texttt{mid} + \beta_3\texttt{high}$$

has an inherent ambiguity.

Specifically, this model specifies every city has a mean temperature of

$$\alpha + \beta_1$$

for sea-level cities,

$$\alpha + \beta_2$$

for medium-altitude cities, or else

$$\alpha + \beta_3$$

for high-altitude cities.

The problem is there are three types of cities, but the model expresses this in four parameter values. There is no unique value we can assign to the intercept α, for example. We might set $\alpha = 0$ and have each of the βs equal to the mean for the respective group of cities. We could just as well set the intercept equal to 1 and then set all of the βs equal to 1 less than the averages of the three groups. In this manner, we could assign any value to the intercept. **R** will be unable to fit the model and will (arbitrarily) set β_3 equal to zero.

Such a model is said to suffer from *multicolinearity* or to be *not of full rank*. In multicolinearity, there exists a linear relationship between some of the explanatory variables.

To identify the source of the problem, in the example with the three categories of cities, we note every city has to be in one of the three categories. If we know two of the indicator values for any given city, then we can immediately determine the value of the third. The three indicator variables always sum to one, so

$$\texttt{sea} + \texttt{mid} + \texttt{high} = 1$$

for every city resulting in the multicolinearity.

In the case of these three categorical indicators, we can use at most two in a linear regression. The use of all three will cause multicolinearity. Notice also, in the previous example of northern and southern cities, there was only one indicator variable in the model for the two categories. In that example, we used an indicator for northern cities but our model did not also include the complementary indicator for southern cities.

How many indicators should be used? The rule is as follows.

Use one fewer indicators than categories in your model.

If we try to fit a model with one indicator variable for every category, then the model will suffer from multicolinearity. We need to leave at least one out of the model.

Having said this, which altitude indicator should we omit? The answer to this question depends on how we want to interpret the fitted regression coefficients. The omitted indicator becomes the *reference category* because it is associated with the intercept. In most regression models, the intercept is not always useful, as we saw in the exercise of Section 5.7.2.

In the present example, let us illustrate the use of a reference category by omitting the indicator for sea-level cities. The **R** code in Output 6.3 fits the model

$$\texttt{JanT} = \alpha + \beta_1\,\texttt{mid} + \beta_2\,\texttt{high}.$$

For sea-level cities, both $\texttt{mid}$ and $\texttt{high}$ are equal to zero, so the average January temperature is equal to the estimated intercept 52.96. The estimated regression coefficients on $\texttt{mid}$ and $\texttt{high}$ correspond to differences from the average of the-sea level cities, as we see next. This motivates the description of sea level as being the reference category.

For cities between 100 and 1000 feet above sea level, the $\texttt{mid}$ indicator is equal to 1 and $\texttt{high}$ is equal to 0. The average January temperature for such cities is then estimated as

$$52.96 - 13.61 = 38.35,$$

where -13.61 is the estimated regression coefficient for $\texttt{mid}$ given in Output 6.3.

The estimated regression coefficient -13.61 for $\texttt{mid}$ is significantly different from zero with a p-value of 0.001. This indicates such cities are significantly colder than sea-level cities, in line with our intuition.

Output 6.3 **R** output for the three categories of altitude.

```
            > alt.reg <- lm(city$JanT ~ mid + high, data = city)
> summary(alt.reg)


Call:
lm(formula = city$JanT ~ mid + high, data = city)

Residuals:
    Min     1Q  Median     3Q     Max
-21.956  -9.348  -2.867   9.043  29.044

Coefficients:
             Estimate Std. Error t value Pr(>|t|)
(Intercept)    51.957      2.787  18.640  < 2e-16 ***
mid           -13.609      3.942  -3.452  0.00104 **
high          -12.090      4.436  -2.725  0.00848 **
---
Signif. codes:  0 '***' 0.001 '**' 0.01 '*' 0.05 '.' 0.1 ' ' 1

Residual standard error: 13.37 on 58 degrees of freedom
Multiple R-squared:  0.1909, Adjusted R-squared:  0.163
F-statistic: 6.844 on 2 and 58 DF,  p-value: 0.002146
```

For cities above 1000 feet, we estimate the maximum January temperature to be

$$51.96 - 12.09 = 39.87,$$

where -12.09 is the estimated regression coefficient for high in Output 6.3. The estimated coefficient -12.09 is the difference in average temperature between sea level and high altitude cities.

As with middle-altitude cities, the regression coefficient for high-altitude cities compares these to the cities at sea level. This illustrates how the omitted indicator variable defines the reference category. The estimated regression coefficients of mid and high correspond to differences with the sea-level cities, justifying our description of sea as the reference category.

What is not intuitive is high-altitude cities are estimated to be *warmer* than mid-altitude cities. This is counter to our understanding of these data. After all, from the estimated regression coefficient on Alt in Output 5.1, we see cities at higher altitude are supposed to be colder.

The explanation of this curious conclusion is cities at higher altitude generally are cooler, but this relationship is not linear. If we only looked at the output of Table 5.1, then we might be led to believe cities at higher altitudes are colder at a constant change in temperature per foot above sea level.

A quick examination, however, of the scatter plot of maximum January temperature by altitude in the extreme upper right-hand corner of Fig. 5.1 shows this relationship is not linear at all. One problem is cities are not evenly distributed across altitudes and climates. The sea-level cities experience a very wide range of climates but the few, influential, highest-altitude cities are colder than average. From the estimated regression coefficients in Output 6.3, we see much of the drop in average temperature occurs between sea-level and mid-altitude cities. The difference in average temperature between mid-altitude and high-altitude cities is small. See Exercise 6.2 for more discussion on this.

If the use of a single indicator variable (such as DC) in a regression model mimics the t-test, then what is the analogous interpretation of several indicators, such as `sea`, `mid`, and `high`? This generalization of the t-test to comparisons of several groups is called a *one-way* ANOVA. There are often settings where more than two groups of data values need to be compared. Another example involving a comparison of three groups is given in Table 7.5 in Chapter 7. Exercise 6.5 examines the assumptions of the one-way ANOVA. A method to perform the one-way ANOVA is described in Exercise 7.8.

In this section, we have seen that linear regression can sometimes be more than we really need. Indicator variables can provide us with a simplified description of the data if we use them carefully and then interpret the results. An easily remembered rule about altitude can be helpful in a recipe and also when explaining temperatures. When it comes time to explain a complicated data set, your audience will often appreciate simplicity rather than a surfeit of precision.

When we omitted the indicator for sea-level cities, these became the intercept or the reference category. The indicator variables remaining in the model acts as comparisons with the reference because their estimated regression coefficients are differences of averages with the reference category. Specifically, in Output 6.3 we see the intercept is the average temperature of sea-level cities. The regression slopes on `mid` and `high` are the differences in average temperatures between mid-altitude and high-altitude cities, respectively, and the cities at sea level.

> The category of the omitted indicator becomes the reference. Estimated regression slopes are differences of averages with this reference.

In Section 6.3 we will see that indicator variables can be combined with other variables. These techniques have useful interpretations as well when we want to measure synergy. Before we go there, Section 6.2 illustrates how two different drugs can be combined, resulting in a greater or lower effect than what we might have expected from their individual contributions.

6.2   Drug Interactions

The interaction of two or more drugs is usually interpreted to mean an unintended side-effect. Here we examine a drug interaction resulting in a greater (or lower) effect than we would anticipate from their individual effects. This section summarizes a study of interactions of anti-fungal drugs in inhibiting cell growth in a single-celled yeast. The uses of this yeast were known in ancient times. Today, it is frequently used in baking bread, brewing beer, and making wine, for example.

By combining pairs of anti-fungal drugs at different concentrations, the article demonstrates how the drugs inhibit cell growth. This reduction in cell growth may equal the sum of their individual effects, acting independently. Similarly, this growth may be greater than or less than the sum of their individual effects. The authors of the article refer to these interaction effects as *synergy* and *antagonism*, respectively, depending on whether the two drugs appear to enhance their actions or work against each other.

Figure 6.1 illustrates the basic experiment and how the data is displayed. A pair of drugs are called A and B in Fig. 6.1 (a). Both drugs are combined at each of eight different levels chosen between zero and their respective minimal inhibitory concentration (MIC). Yeast is grown under each of these 64 experimental conditions. These 64 experimental combinations are summarized in Fig. 6.1 (b) as shaded grids with lighter shades indicating greater cell grown, and darker shades corresponding to lower or no growth. In the lower-left corner, with neither drug present, we see white,

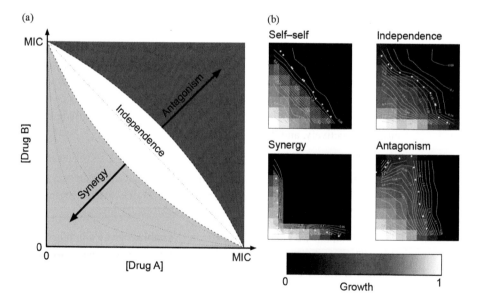

Figure 6.1 Graphical depiction of the interactions of two drugs: (a) idealized and (b) four examples of actual data.
Source: Cokol M, Chua HN, Tasan M *et al.* (2011).

or the maximum possible level of growth corresponding to zero levels of both drugs. Each of the four parts of Fig. 6.1 (b) grows darker toward the upper-right indicating greater cell-growth inhibition.

Each of the four plots in Fig. 6.1 (b) includes estimated contour levels of conditions exhibiting identical rates of cell growth. These are similar to the temperature contours appearing in the weather map, Fig. 1.1.

If a drug is matched with itself (labeled *self–self* in the figure) then these contours are almost parallel lines running upper-left to lower-right. A similar set of contours appear if the two drugs act independently.

If the drugs exhibit synergism then these contours bend inward toward the lower left corner. That is, if the two drug effects reinforce each other (synergism), then small amounts of both will achieve a much greater inhibition of cell growth than an equivalent amount of either one alone. Conversely, if the drugs work against each other (antagonism), then the contours will bulge out toward the upper right indicating a much greater level of cell growth than achieved by one drug alone.

Figure 6.2 displays the full set of plots for all pairs of 13 anti-fungal drugs studied. Every drug is identified by a three-letter abbreviation. Each drug is matched with itself and all 12 others and is presented as matrix, much as the scatter plot in Fig. 2.13.

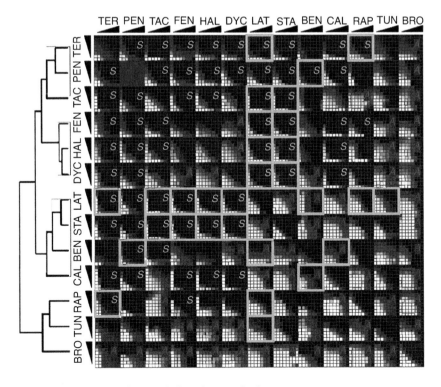

Figure 6.2 Synergistic display of all 13 drugs, paired.

Each combination pair is classified as either synergistic or antagonistic with an S or an A, respectively. Briefly, we can see drug combinations with a lot of white space having high cell growth and classified as antagonistic. Similarly, combinations with a lot of dark space have low cell growth and are synergistic. On the left side of Fig. 6.2, there is a tree figure illustrating the proximity of effect for each drug to the others.

A lot of work went into collecting the data for this experiment and then displaying it in a thoughtful manner.

In Section 6.3, we return to indicator variables and use these to study synergism in linear models. Briefly, we examine whether the net effect of two variables is greater than, less than, or equal to the sum of their individual contributions.

6.3   Interactions of Explanatory Variables

Northern cities are colder than average, as are cities situated at high altitude. What can we say about northern cities at high altitude? Are these even colder than expected? What is the combined effect of altitude and latitude?

We can measure the combined or synergistic effects by creating additional indicator variables. In Section 6.1, we created the indicator DC for northern cities and mid and high for medium- and high-altitude cities. We can create indicators for the combined effects of high altitude and northern latitude by creating an indicator variable equal to 1 for cities having both attributes. An easy way to do this is by multiplying these separate indicators together to form new indicators.

If we add the lines

```
hinorth <- DC * high
midnorth <- DC * mid
seanorth <- DC * sea
```

then we have created indicators of these interaction effects.

As an example of this coding, hinorth is equal to 1 for cities both at high altitude and located north of Washington but equal to 0 for other cities.

In Section 6.1, we saw the temperatures of sea-level cities are different from those at medium and high altitudes. In Fig. 5.1 we saw a large amount of climate variability among the sea-level cities. Perhaps we can use the seanorth indicator variable to separate and explain some of this variation in the cities situated at or near sea level. As an example, seanorth is equal to 1 for sea-level cities north of Washington but 0 for all other cities.

> An interaction variable is constructed as the
> product of any two explanatory variables.

These three interactions can be included with other indicators in a model statement as follows.

```
lm( JanT ~ DC + high + sea + hinorth + seanorth, data = city)
```

Recall the discussion of multicolinearity in Section 6.1. In this program, we cannot include the three indicators for altitude: sea, mid, and high. In this present example we chose to omit the middle category of altitude. Similarly, we cannot fit a model with all three interactions of altitude and north/south, because the sum of these three will be the same as the DC indicator variable. Again, we chose to omit the middle interaction denoted by midnorth, and this will define our reference category.

This regression model contains two types of indicators: those for the north/south cities (DC) and for altitude; and those making up the interactions (hinorth and seanorth). Terms such as DC and high and sea are usually referred to as *main effects* in the model, because the interactions are products of these. It is good statistical practice to include the main effects of all interactions in order to facilitate their interpretation. Without both of the main effects in the model, the interaction would model a combination of both the underlying main effect and the interaction. As a result, such an interaction could be difficult to interpret.

Output 6.4 **R** program with interactions in the January temperature data.

```
> hinorth <- DC * high
> midnorth <- DC * mid
> seanorth <- DC * sea
>
> interact <- lm( JanT  ~  DC + high + sea + hinorth + seanorth, data = city)
> summary(interact)

Call:
lm(formula = JanT ~ DC + high + sea + hinorth + seanorth, data = city)

Residuals:
    Min      1Q  Median      3Q     Max
-20.417  -4.111  -0.375   4.636  16.583

Coefficients:
             Estimate Std. Error t value Pr(>|t|)
(Intercept)    51.375      2.763  18.592  < 2e-16 ***
DCTRUE        -19.975      3.422  -5.838 2.94e-07 ***
high           -1.375      4.221  -0.326 0.745851
sea            13.042      3.567   3.656 0.000574 ***
hinorth         3.086      5.355   0.576 0.566769
seanorth       -6.078      4.728  -1.286 0.203976
---
Signif. codes:  0 '***' 0.001 '**' 0.01 '*' 0.05 '.' 0.1 ' ' 1

Residual standard error: 7.816 on 55 degrees of freedom
Multiple R-squared:  0.7377, Adjusted R-squared:  0.7139
F-statistic: 30.94 on 5 and 55 DF,  p-value: 7.774e-15
```

Table 6.2 Model parameters for the six different types of cities.

City location		
Latitude	Altitude	Parameters in model
South of DC	Sea level	$\alpha + \beta_{\text{sea}}$
South of DC	Mid-altitude	α
South of DC	High altitude	$\alpha + \beta_{\text{hi}}$
North of DC	Sea level	$\alpha + \beta_{\text{DC}} + \beta_{\text{sea}} + \beta_{\text{seaN}}$
North of DC	Mid-altitude	$\alpha + \beta_{\text{DC}}$
North of DC	High altitude	$\alpha + \beta_{\text{DC}} + \beta_{\text{hi}} + \beta_{\text{hiN}}$

A portion of the output from this program is contained in Output 6.4. The largest effect is for latitude, and cities north of Washington are estimated to be more than 19 degrees colder than those to the south. We omitted the indicator for mid-altitude, southern cities and, as a result, these cities correspond to the intercept of the model. Before we try to interpret the values in Output 6.4, it is useful to write out the parameters of the model and see how they fit together.

The fitted model is

$$\texttt{maxt} = \alpha + \beta_{\text{DC}}\,\texttt{DC} + \beta_{\text{hi}}\,\texttt{high} + \beta_{\text{sea}}\,\texttt{sea}$$
$$+ \beta_{\text{hiN}}\,\texttt{hinorth} + \beta_{\text{seaN}}\,\texttt{seanorth}.$$

The estimated regression coefficients appear in Output 6.4. In order to interpret these, we first write out which parameters go with which cities. This is given in Table 6.2.

There are a total of six types of cities being modeled: north or south and three categories of altitudes (sea level, and mid- and high-altitude). The intercept α appears in the model for all six city types. We omitted indicators for southern cities and mid-altitude cities, so this type of city becomes the reference category. Specifically, we see the intercept alone appears in the model for southern, mid-altitude cities.

All southern cities have $\texttt{DC} = 0$, so the regression coefficient β_{DC} only appears in the three categories of northern cities. Similarly, $\texttt{sea} = 1$ only for sea-level cities and β_{sea} appears only in models for sea-level cities. The main effect for high altitude and its regression coefficient β_{hi} only appears in the model for high-altitude cities.

By way of interpretation of these main effects, we can say they *correct* for the effects of latitude and altitude. These main effects suggest the maximum January temperature of each of the six groups of cities can be expressed as a latitude effect (north or south of Washington) plus an effect due to altitude (in one of three categories). That is, we are expressing the average maximum January temperature as

$$\text{Maximum January temperature} = \text{Latitude effect} + \text{Altitude effect}, \qquad (6.1)$$

or as the sums of its two component parts.

The estimated coefficient for $\texttt{high}$ is -1.375 and is not statistically different from zero. Consequently, we conclude cities at high altitude are not significantly colder than cities at mid-altitude. This conclusion is consistent with the fitted model we saw in

Output 6.3. Cities at sea level are much warmer than mid-altitude cities. The estimated regression coefficient on sea is 13.0 and is statistically significant. Perhaps we can simplify the altitude effect into two component values: near sea level and more than 100 feet above sea level, because there appears to be negligible difference between mid-altitude and high-altitude cities.

Interactions are concerned with exceptions to the model (6.1). The interaction called seanorth is only equal to 1 when the city is located both in the north and at sea level. The corresponding regression coefficient β_{seaN} only appears in the model for such cities. Similarly, the interaction hinorth is only equal to 1 for high-altitude, northern cities. The corresponding parameter β_{hiN} only appears in Table 6.2 for such cities.

When we look at the estimated interactions in Output 6.4, we see sea-level cities in the north are 6.1 degrees colder than we would expect them to be based only on a model with main effects. These main effects include the separate effects of being in the north and being at sea level. Without these two main effects, it would be difficult to interpret the estimated regression coefficient of seanorth in this model. The regression coefficient for this interaction is not statistically significant, but we see these cities are colder than expected. Similarly, northern cities at high altitudes are not statistically colder than expected. In fact, such cities are estimated to be about 3.1 degrees warmer than expected, after including the separate main effects of being at high altitude and being located in the northern half of the country.

Let us make one final point for this example. In Output 6.4, we see the estimated effect of being located north of Washington is estimated as 19.975 degrees colder, on average, than cities south of Washington. In Output 6.1 of the previous section this effect is measured to be −23.05. Although these two estimates are close and are both negative, as we would expect, how do we account for the difference in values?

The answer is: The indicator variables high and sea are correlated with DC. There is not an even balance of US cities located at different altitudes and latitudes. The effects of the indicators overlap slightly and attempt to measure the same attributes in the data. Recall from Section 5.5 how we tried to measure accurately the effect an infant's length had on its weight. Many of the variables in the low-birth-weight infant data set are mutually correlated, and it is sometimes difficult to distinguish the effects of any one of these on the weight outcome. A similar situation occurs when we create indicators for altitude and latitude. These are also correlated, and their explanatory values overlap in a regression model.

In general, it is a good idea to examine the interactions of variables we find to be statistically significant in our models. If the variables are separately important in explaining the outcome, then their interaction may provide even more value. Interactions are generally harder to find statistically significant because the power to detect them is lower than for the main effects. Always include the original main effects in order to facilitate the interpretation of the regression coefficients. Finally, interactions need not be constructed only from indicator variables. The interaction of any two variables (either continuous or discrete valued) can be constructed as the product of the two.

If you accidentally include variables resulting in multicolinearity, you should be able to recognize the problem. **R** will fit a model by omitting one or more variables to remove the multicolinearity. This choice by **R** may not be what you want and may not result in a model with an easy interpretation. The interpretation of the intercept and reference category will change depending on the omitted category.

6.4   Transformations

Table 6.3 presents the 2005 average price of gasoline (in US dollars) and average daily consumption per person for several different countries.[1] What determines the price: How much it is taxed, the rate of consumption, or whether the country produces and exports oil? Both Norway and Iran export oil, but Iran has very low consumption per person. Norway has higher consumption and also very high taxes on gasoline. The economy of Singapore relies heavily on shipping and the petrochemical industry, including refining; all of these consume a lot of oil. Given the data in this table, how can we make a convincing argument that per-person consumption plays a role in the price of gasoline?

The graph in Fig. 6.3 (a) plots the raw data including the fitted regression line. The slope of this line is 0.22 with an estimated standard error of 0.30. (See Exercise 6.7

Table 6.3 The price of a gallon of gasoline and the average daily consumption per person in selected countries.

Country	Price in US dollars	Consumption per person
Norway	6.66	1.9
Netherlands	6.55	2.3
Britain	6.17	1.2
Germany	5.98	1.4
Italy	5.94	1.4
France	5.68	1.4
Singapore	3.50	7.3
Brazil	3.35	0.5
India	3.29	0.1
Mexico	3.20	0.8
South Africa	3.13	0.4
United States	2.26	2.9
Russia	2.05	0.8
China	1.78	0.2
Nigeria	1.48	0.1
Iran	0.47	0.8

Source: Reuters; Energy Information Administration.

[1] Also available online at www.nytimes.com/2005/04/30/business/worldbusiness/30norway.html.

(a) Price in $

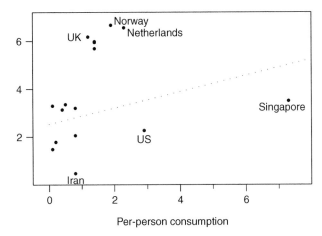

(b) Logarithm of consumption

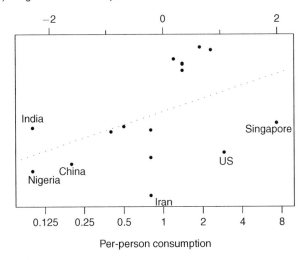

Figure 6.3 Observed data and fitted regressions of gasoline price using consumption and log consumption.

for more on interpreting this slope.) The statistical significance level is $p = 0.49$, indicating a weak linear relationship between price and consumption. In Fig. 6.3 (a) we see Singapore has a large influence in this regression model because its consumption is so much greater than that of any other country in the data set. A number of low-price and low-consumption nations (including Iran) are clustered in a tight bunch at the lower left of this figure. It is not clear whether a linear regression is even appropriate from this scatter plot.

Instead of examining per person consumption, suppose we examine the log (base e) of consumption. This is a new variable created by inserting the line

```
logcon <- log(consume)
```

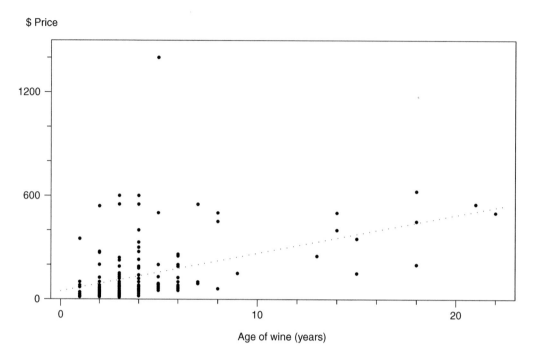

$ Price

Figure 6.4 Wine price by age and the fitted regression line.

into the **R** program. Again, we should remember to print out the data to check our work.

The graph in Fig. 6.3 (b) shows this log transformation spreads apart the data on the group of low-consumption and low-gasoline-price countries. We are able to identify the data values for India, Nigeria, and China, for example. This log transformation also pulls in the observation for Singapore and makes it much less influential in the fitted regression. The log consumption values used in the linear regression are listed along the top of the figure. The values on the original scale are listed at the bottom.

The slope for this new fitted regression on log consumption is 0.79 with a standard error of 0.41 and statistical significance $p = 0.07$. (See Exercise 6.7 for interpreting this slope.) This improved statistical significance provides a better measure of the effect consumption has on the price of gasoline. The overall regression influence is more evenly spread among all nations in the data set after we take the logarithm of the consumption values.

> The logarithm transformation of a variable will pull in large
> values and spread apart the low values.

Let us consider another example of transformations in regression. Table 5.5 lists the prices of wine in an advertisement. In this example we want to examine the relationship between the age and the price of the wine.

A scatter plot of price by age is given in Fig. 6.4. In this figure, we cannot see much, if any, relationship between these two variables. The prices are mostly bunched up in the lower left corner. There is one extreme price near the top. Many of the wines are fairly new, but there are a few older than 10 years. The vertical stripes occur because vintage years are discrete valued. Sometimes jittering the age values can help the display in a figure like this.

The linear regression is statistically significant and $R^2 = 0.2$. The estimated slope is about 22, indicating the wine appreciates at \$22 per year. The relatively small value of R^2 and this figure does not provide very convincing evidence of a linear relationship between wine price and its age. The exercise of Section 6.6.1 asks you to see how much influence the very oldest wines contribute to the linear regression.

In Fig. 6.3 we saw taking logarithms of the gasoline consumption values pulled apart the group of tightly-clustered low values and also reduced the effect of the extremely high values.

Let us try this with the wine data. In Fig. 6.5, we see taking logs of price has a similar effect. A price in log-dollars may not make sense to most people, so it often helps to include the axis on the right side of this figure, which provides the corresponding values in dollar amounts. Recall the log scale is multiplicative, so the distance from 25 to 50 is the same as from 50 to 100 and the same as from 250 to 500.

The effect of taking logs of price is to break up the tight cluster of values in the lower left corner of the original data plotted in Fig. 6.4. By taking logs of price, we can more clearly see individual data points in Fig. 6.5. The one very high priced \$1400 wine is no longer such an extreme outlier.

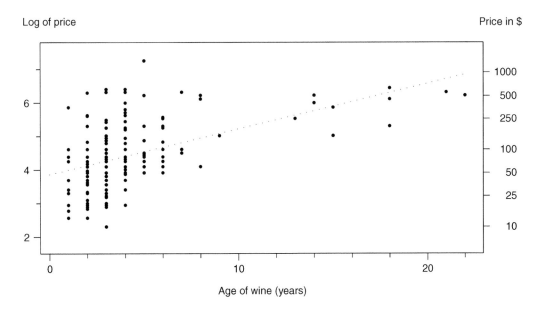

Figure 6.5 Log of wine price by age and the fitted regression line.

The linear regression on log price has an improved $R^2 = 0.245$, as well. Wines younger than 10 years have a wide range of prices. Wines older than 10 years have a smaller variation in relative price. These older wines are more expensive than the average younger wines, but this difference is not dramatic. This difference is probably the largest contributor to the statistical significance of the fitted regression model. See Section 6.6.1 for an examination of this claim.

This regression has a slope of 0.136. Taking logs of the response variable puts the regression on a multiplicative scale. Comparing one year to the next, this model suggests prices will be in the ratio of

$$\exp(0.136) = 1.146$$

to 1. That is to say, this model estimates, on average, these wine prices will increase by 14.6% for every year of age.

In Fig. 6.5, we also see the older wines are separated from the others along the age axis, and a few of these influential observations are older than 10 years. We can take logs of the age values as well as price. This is plotted in Fig. 6.6. As with the price values, it is often helpful to your reader if you provide the actual values rather than the transformed values.

In Fig. 6.6, we can see the age values more evenly spread out, without the oldest ages exerting great influence. The linear regression in this figure has $R^2 = 0.27$, and the figure provides good evidence of a linear fit to the data. There are no apparent outliers on the log-price scale, and the oldest ages, also on a log scale, are not influential. There appears to be larger variation in price at younger ages than among the older wines, but otherwise this appears to be a good application of linear regression.

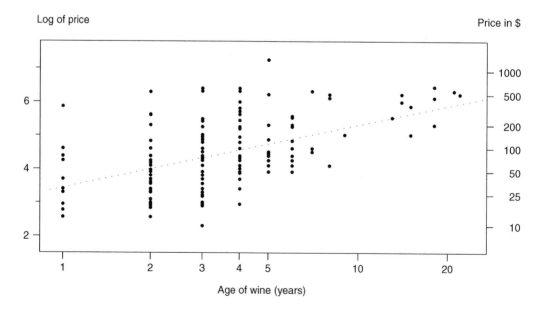

Figure 6.6 Wine price by age, both on a log scale, and the fitted regression line.

The estimated regression slope for the transformed data in Fig. 6.6 is 0.812. Both price and age are measured on a log scale, so both have to be interpreted in a multiplicative fashion. Specifically, the estimated ratio of the average price of one wine is

$$2^{0.812} = 1.756$$

times as great as the price of another wine with half the age. At twice the age, then, a wine should cost 75.6% greater, on average.

In this section, the two examples demonstrated that taking logs may sometimes remove influence and reduce the appearance of outliers. Logarithms also pulled apart tight clusters of data points, allowing these to be more clearly seen and to contribute equally to the fitted regression model. Exercise 6.1 provides another example of this.

The square-root transformation may also be used. The square-root transformation is not as extreme as the logarithm and has a more subtle effect. See Exercise 6.3 for an example of this.

There are other important instances in which we might want to transform one or more variables in a linear regression. Sometimes the scatter plot suggests the data are related, but not in a linear fashion. In the exercise of Section 6.6.4, we examine tumor growth rates in mice. These sometimes grow at an exponential rate and a log transformation may be appropriate in order to apply a linear regression model. In other settings we might accept the nonlinear relationship and try to model it. In Exercise 6.6.8 we describe how to fit a nonlinear relationship with a model containing both the explanatory variable and the square of this variable.

6.5   Additional Topics: Longitudinal Data

As part of a survey conducted by Pew,[2] Table 6.4 summarizes the attitudes toward the United States held by citizens of several other countries at up to five different time points. What is the best way to use regression to analyze this data?

Longitudinal data is the study of observations where a change is only apparent over a period of observation. In this example, different people were surveyed at two or more different times. This is sometimes called *panel data*, in which a cross-section of the population is examined. This is how public health data might be summarized by reporting the responses of all persons surveyed, over time.

Similarly, we might ask how individual countries' attitudes change. Such a study is called *transitional* or how responses at one time are related to those in the same individual at a later date.

In medical studies, we might follow and collect data on the same subject over time. We might ask whether individuals with poor initial conditions improve during this interval. This is the transitional approach to examining longitudinal data. Random effects models (see also Section 6.6.4) are useful for this type of modeling, where every subject is measured several times. In public health, we might ask whether the

---

[2] Availale online at http://people-press.org/reports/pdf/185.pdf.

Table 6.4 Percentage favorable attitudes toward the United States by country.

	1999–2000	Summer 2002	March 2003	June 2003	2019
Israel	–	–	–	79	81
Great Britain	83	75	48	70	57
Kuwait	–	–	–	63	
Canada	71	72	–	63	51
Nigeria	46	77	–	61	62
Australia	–	–	–	60	50
Italy	76	70	34	60	62
South Korea	58	53	–	46	77
Germany	78	61	25	45	39
France	62	63	31	43	46
Spain	50	–	14	38	52
Russia	37	61	28	36	29
Brazil	56	52	–	34	56
Morocco	77	–	–	27	
Lebanon	–	35	–	27	39
Indonesia	75	61	–	15	42
Turkey	52	30	12	15	20
Pakistan	23	10	–	13	
Jordan	–	25	–	1	
Palestian Auth.	14	–	–	1	

Source: Pew Research Center.

average for the whole population changes at each time point. This is the marginal approach. An analysis of the longitudinal data in Table 6.4 is given in Exercise 6.6. Another examination of longitudinal data appears in Exercise 9.4.2.

One of the difficulties occurring when subjects are measured more than once is called *regression to the mean*. Suppose there was no difference in attitudes between the various countries at two different time points. In this case, we would expect those surveys more favorable than average at the first interview time would tend to be more like the average on the second survey. Similarly, those most unfavorable at the time of the first interview should look more favorable at the next survey. This property is called regression to the mean, because extremes above and below the average will look more like the average when measured a second time. An example of this behavior is examined in Exercise 6.4.

Another difficulty with longitudinal data is the presence of missing data. Missing data is very common in longitudinal medical and social data, where subjects are asked to return for periodic reexaminations. There can be many reasons for missing data. As an example, did individuals with extreme attitudes refuse to answer the US attitude survey? In this case there would be a bias in the observed data, because whether or not a data point was missing would be related to what its value might have been had it been observed.

One quick fix for missing data in longitudinal surveys is to use the last observed value. This approach of *last observed value carried forward* is a simple and well-accepted approach to filling in most of the missing values in a longitudinal survey. Clearly this technique would not work for Israel, Kuwait, or Australia which have no earlier observations, but many of the other missing values in this table could be replaced in this manner. Another popular method for filling in missing values is called the *hot deck* in which we use the observed value of the last individual who is similar to the one with missing values.

6.6   Exercises

6.1 Notice how skewed the altitude values are in Fig. 5.1. Plot the `dfbeta` for altitude and then again in the model with log altitude. Does this logarithmic transformation reduce the influence of cities at the highest altitudes?

6.2 Examine the three indicator variables for city altitude described in Section 6.1. Use indicator variables in linear regression to show the difference in maximum January temperature between medium-altitude and high-altitude cities is not statistically significant. Hint: Use either the mid- or high-altitude cities as the reference category.

6.3 Reexamine the gasoline consumption data of Table 6.3. Consider the square root of the consumption values. This is done by creating a new variable in the data step using the `sqrt` function in **R**. Specifically, the line in the program might look like the following.

```
sqcons   <- sqrt(consume)
```

Does this transformation provide a better linear regression than the original data? Look at the hat matrix diagonals to see if the highest-consuming countries are as influential as they were in the original data. Compare the square-root transformation to the log transformation for these data. Which of these two depictions of the data do your prefer?

6.4 We asked a room full of statistics students to predict the order in which heads and tails appear after 10 successive tosses of a coin. Some people were very good at this and took the rest of the day off. Those who lacked this skill were required to watch a movie about how coins are minted and then review Section 2.1 on the binomial distribution. This must have been a good strategy, because the next day, the former poor predictors did much better, on average. Unfortunately, however, those who took the afternoon off failed to do as well as they did the day before. What happened?

6.5 The one-way ANOVA is the generalization of the t-test to more than two groups of subjects. This is described at the end of Section 6.1, comparing cities at one of three different altitudes. In general, what assumptions of Section 4.4 need to be met when we perform a one-way ANOVA?

6.6 a. Consider a marginal analysis of the attitude survey given in Table 6.4. We can perform a t-test to compare the mean attitude at the time of any two surveys. Each of the countries is compared at two different times, so we should perform a *paired t-test*. The paired t-test is the same as a one-sample t-test performed on the column of difference values. We want to test the null hypothesis the mean difference is equal to 0. Is there a downward trend in the means? Is there evidence the survey favored countries with a higher initial attitude?

b. There are several different ways to perform a transitional analysis. We might begin by plotting the attitude values (on the vertical scale) against time of the survey and drawing a line connecting the values for the same country. This mix of lines is called a *spaghetti plot* for obvious reasons. Spaghetti plots will often reveal the general trend of the individuals. Construct the spaghetti plot for the data in Table 6.4. In this figure, do the low initial attitudes tend to become lower in the later survey, or are these more likely to increase? That is, does there appear to be a regression to the mean? What can be said about countries with high initial attitudes toward the United States?

c. What is gained by filling in the missing values of a longitudinal study? Should these be treated as actual, observed values when the data is analyzed?

6.7 The estimated slope of the data in Fig. 6.3 (a) is 0.22. Interpret this value. If consumption is measured on a log scale then the estimated slope is 0.79. Show, if consumption is doubled, this model estimates the price per person should increase $0.79 \log(2) = \$0.55$ per person, on average.

6.6.1   More on Wine Prices

Let us reexamine the wine price exercise of Section 5.7.5. We can make use of methods described in this chapter, specifically, transformations and interactions of variables. The data is given in Table 5.5.

a. Examine the difference in prices between wines older and younger than 10 years using a t-test. Compare the results if price is measured on a log scale or a linear scale. Which comparison seems more appropriate?

b. How do the experts' points relate to price? Is there a benefit in transforming the points as well as price values?

c. Repeat some of the analysis performed in Section 5.7.5 for these data using transformed values. Do you identify the same wines as bargains or overpriced you identified in the earlier examination of this data?

d. Is there a synergistic interaction between experts' points and old vintage when it comes to modeling the price of a wine? That is, do old wines with high points command a much higher premium than what we might expect from these two factors separately?

Table 6.5 Cigarette brands and their nicotine content.

Brand	Menthol?	Length	Filtered?	Manufacturer	Nicotine
Old Gold		85	nonfilter	Lorillard	4.1
Max		120	filter	Lorillard	3.4
Newport	M	100	filter	Lorillard	3.2
Camel		70	nonfilter	RJ Reynolds	3.0
Doral		85	nonfilter	RJ Reunolds	3.0
Newport	M	85	filter	Lorillard	2.8
Maverick	M	100	filter	Lorillard	2.7
Camel		100	filter	RJ Reynolds	2.6
Maverick		100	filter	Lorillard	2.5
Kool	M	100	filter	RJ Reynolds	2.5
Newport		100	filter	Lorillard	2.5
Marlboro		100	filter	Phillip Morris	2.4

Source: Massachusetts Department of Public Health.

6.6.2   Nicotine Levels in Cigarettes

Table 6.5 presents data on the cigarettes with the highest nicotine content. A number of comparisons can be made. For example, we can statistically compare the nicotine contents of Lorillard versus all other manufacturers, menthol versus nonmenthol cigarettes, and filter versus nonfilter brands. These can be done using separate t-tests. A better analysis plan is to create a series of 0–1 indicators and use these simultaneously in the same regression model. How do these simultaneous comparisons provide different explanations from running three separate t-tests?

Examine the interactions among the three indicator variables. How do you interpret these? Should the nicotine levels be transformed? Apply other lessons from this and the previous chapter. Look for influence and outliers. Not every interaction can be estimated because of the imbalance of effects: All menthol cigarettes are also filtered and all but one menthol brand is manufactured by Lorillard.

6.6.3   The Speed of a Reaction

The data in Table 6.6 provides a summary of experiments measuring the speed of an enzymatic reaction both with and without addition of the enzyme puromycin. The reaction depends on the initial concentration (in parts per million), and its rate is measured in radioactive counts per minute.

Plot the rate (y) as a function of initial concentration (x) and describe the relationship. The authors of these data had theoretical evidence for a specific nonlinear relationship between these variables. Try a log or square-root transformation of the rate. Does this produce a better linear relationship?

What effect does addition of puromycin have on the rate of the reaction? Propose a model and fit it. After transforming the rate, is there evidence of a nonconstant variance? Are there outliers to be pointed out?

Table 6.6 Data on the speed of an enzymatic reaction both with and without addition of the enzyme puromycin.

Initial concentration	Rate	Puromycin?
0.02	76	treated
0.02	47	treated
0.06	97	treated
⋮		
0.56	144	untreated
0.56	158	untreated
1.10	160	untreated

Available as data(Puromycin) in **R**.

Table 6.7 Tumor volumes (in mm³) in 10 mice.

	Days after injection			
Mouse #	11	13	15	17
1	157.1	217.6	379.0	556.6
2	152.2	176.6	317.9	356.4
3	122.4	196.1	388.9	496.3
4	95.0	205.9	307.3	405.1
5	168.8	196.0	340.4	507.3
6	85.0	225.1	289.0	317.9
7	129.8	274.7	340.3	507.2
8	157.0	202.5	307.2	320.1
9	129.7	205.8	419.1	421.2
10	156.9	225.0	372.6	379.2

Source: Koziol *et al.* (1981).

## 6.6.4	Tumor Growth in Mice

In a commonly conducted experiment, a small piece of a human tumor is injected under the skin of a mouse. If the tumor successfully implants and continues to grow, a palpable lump will be felt under the mouse's skin. The volume of this lump can be measured, and changes in its size over time are indicative of the virulence of the tumor. An example of such an experiment is given in Table 6.7 for 10 mice.

Draw the spaghetti plot for these data. Perform a linear regression modeling tumor size by date for these 10 mice. Check the residuals of this model. Does the regression look linear? Try jittering the dates in the graph to improve the appearance. Of course, you don't want to jitter the dates you use in the regression model.

Consider a log transformation of the size values. Does this improve the linearity of the model? Taking logs is a reasonable approach if you think tumor growth is exponential in time. What is wrong with assuming the exponential growth will continue?

Notice every mouse is measured four times. Is the linear regression approach valid? Recall the four assumptions we made about linear regression in Section 4.4. One approach taking into account the multiple observations on the same individual is called *random effects*.

In a random effects model, we might assume every mouse has its own intercept and slope, but collectively all these intercepts and slopes are not very different from each other. Biologically, each individual intercept and slope may depend on each of the experimental conditions experienced by each mouse, such as the size of the tumor injected or differences in the way it was injected. Random effects models for longitudinal data are described in Section 6.5. Is there evidence the slopes or intercepts are very different for each mouse?

6.6.5   Used Car Prices

Table 6.8 gives the prices of used Mercedes in an advertisement from a car dealer. For each car, we have the year, class, color, mileage (in thousands of miles) and price (in thousands of dollars). Mercedes produces various models grouped together into larger classes. Cars are listed with two or more colors, and the color listed here is the first color mentioned. Grey includes silver, tan, and pewter; black includes charcoal.

Show marginally, across all model classes, the year is very important in determining the price, but the mileage is not. How do you explain this? Interpret the slope of the year in this regression.

Table 6.8 Prices of used cars from an advertisement appearing in the *New York Times* on August 5, 2007.

Year	Class	Color	Mileage	Price	Year	Class	Color	Mileage	Price
04	E	black	22	30	04	E	grey	25	32
05	E	black	28	34	04	E	blue	35	36
04	E	grey	19	37	05	E	grey	18	40
05	E	grey	30	42	05	E	grey	16	48
05	E	black	40	57	00	S	black	38	30
01	S	grey	17	35	03	S	black	64	36
05	S	grey	36	49	06	S	black	27	53
04	S	grey	14	55	06	S	grey	30	58
06	S	black	18	58	04	S	black	41	62
07	S	blue	12	75	04	CLS	grey	30	53
03	CLS	black	43	58	06	CLS	blue	9	60
04	CLS	blue	32	65	06	CLS	black	20	70
03	CLK	white	35	29	02	CLK	grey	20	32
04	CLK	red	30	33	03	CLK	black	12	36
06	CLK	grey	9	45	04	M	grey	26	28
04	M	grey	13	28	04	M	grey	28	29
05	M	grey	40	30	05	M	grey	23	34
05	M	black	36	34	05	M	grey	20	36
06	M	white	20	39					

When we perform a regression separately for each model class, we see either the year or the model may be statistically significant, sometimes both are, and sometimes neither is. Why do you think this is the case? Notice the intercepts may be either positive or negative in each of these separate regressions. How do you account for this? What does the intercept represent? Is it meaningful?

Is the color important? Create an indicator variable to identify black versus other colors. Use this indicator in your regressions to see if the color of the car influences the price.

Look for outliers and influential observations. Are there bargains or overpriced cars in this dealer's lot? Is there evidence the regression on year is linear? Do these cars appear to depreciate a constant amount every year, or is there evidence the largest depreciation occurs earlier? Which models depreciate faster?

6.6.6   Percent Body Fat

Accurate estimates of total body fat are inconvenient because this involves weighing a subject submersed in a tank of water. The procedure yields a measure of total body density, relative to an equal volume of water. A number of different methods have been suggested over the years to facilitate this computation. Some proposals available include the use of a caliper to measure the thickness of a skin fold. These methods too, have their shortcomings. Can you help find a relatively easy way to measure body fat?

The data includes the body fat measurements of 250 male volunteers, along with a number of other physical attributes. The website

> https://dasl.datadescription.com/datafile/bodyfat/

includes a full explanation of the mathematical relationship between density and body fat often cited, along with many useful references. Another version of the data is available in **R** as BODYFAT in the library regclass with 252 observations. A complete list of the 15 variables measured on each subject is given by typing help("BODYFAT"). There is also a smaller data set is called bodyfat in the **R** library TH.data including several calculated estimates for body fat.

As always, plot the data before you fit models and be on the lookout for outliers. (Hint: There is a 200 pound man who is only 29 inches tall.)

See if you can build a good linear model of percent body fat using any of the regression tools we have learned so far. The percent body fat is computed from underwater density, so your regression model should not include density as an explanatory variable. Some of the physical measurements are highly correlated with each other, and not all may be useful. Be sure to examine your residuals and check for influential observations using diagnostics such as dffits and Cook's D. It is equally acceptable to find a good model to explain density. Percent body fat can be derived from density, so the model for density should not include body fat and vice versa.

Here are some things to look for. Cook's D indicates some very influential observations. One of these is the man with the greatest weight. That observation should be easy to find. The others are not as easy to identify.

In model building we need to make a general statement for most of the population but we must also include provisions for exceptions to the rule. Remember the carnival act in which they guess your weight? Most individuals will follow the general pattern, so this is not as remarkable as it first appears. The real test of the model is to see how general it is. Does it include most of the observed data, or are there many outliers failing to follow the pattern?

6.6.7   Fertility Rates in Switzerland

In 1888, Switzerland began a transition period of reduced birth rates to similar to what they are today. Higher fertility rates before this time are usually associated with those of underdeveloped countries today. This transition is studied by demographers, who note it is associated with the simultaneous rise in life expectancy, drop in birth rate, and rise in incomes. This has led to the *demographic–economic paradox*, in which the richer nations can support more children, yet tend to have lower birth rates. The fertility rate is available in **R** as swiss in the data sets library. A portion of this data is given in Table 6.9.

The columns in the data are:

- the name of the province,
- the standardized fertility rate,
- the percentage of the population with an agricultural occupation,
- the proportion of military draftees who scored high on an army examination,
- the percentage of the population with more than a primary school education,
- the percentage of the population who are Catholic,
- the fraction of births in which the infant does not survive one year.

What are the determinants of the population fertility rate? Model the fertility rates of the different provinces using methods described in this chapter. The percentage of the population with high education, for example, is highly skewed, and the few provinces with high rates have large influence. Try taking logs of the education variable to even out this effect.

Several explanatory variables are correlated with each other. For example, in 1888, agriculture was a labor-intensive effort, and large families were generally more successful. Additional offspring would be needed to offset a high infant mortality.

Table 6.9 A portion of the Swiss fertility rates data.

	Fertility	Agriculture	Examination	Education	Catholic	Infant. Mortality
Courtelary	80.2	17.0	15	12	9.96	2.2
Delemont	83.1	45.1	6	9	84.84	22.2
Franches-Mnt	92.5	39.7	5	5	93.40	20.2
Moutier	85.8	36.5	12	7	33.77	20.3
...						

Table 6.10 A portion of the ELISA data.

Observation number	Run number	Antigen concentration	Optical density
1	1	0.04882812	0.017
2	1	0.04882812	0.018
3	1	0.19531250	0.121
. . .			
176	11	12.50000000	1.721

Lifespans were much shorter than they are today, so higher education was a luxury. Identify any strong relationships between the explanatory variables in your model.

See Exercise 7.9 for additional models of this data. More data from this series as well as other historic demographic data sets are available through the Office of Population Research at Princeton University.[3]

6.6.8   ELISA

ELISA (or enzyme-linked immunosorbent assay) is a technique in biochemistry for detecting an antibody. There are many variants of this popular laboratory method. Briefly, a known concentration of an antigen is put in contact with a serum sample. If there is a match, then the specific antibody will bind to the antigen. This is detected through a change in color or through the use of a fluorescent dye. ELISA is commonly used to detect HIV or West Nile virus, for example. Many ELISA experiments are run simultaneously under identical conditions using an array of small test tubes called *wells*.

The data in Table 6.10 summarizes one such experiment part of the development of an assay for detecting the recombinant protein DNase in rat serum. There were 11 different runs of the experiment. Each run consisted of 8 different concentrations of the antigen, and each of these was replicated for a total of 16 paired observations in each run. The value we want to explain is the optical density.

Plot the concentration on the x axis and the density on the y axis. Does a transformation of the concentration seem appropriate to reduce the influence of higher concentrations? Is there a linear relationship with the optical response? Notice the plot of density by concentration curves in one direction, but the plot with log-concentration curves in the other direction. Consider a model containing both log concentration and the square of log-concentration. Does this improve the fit?

Are there differences in the 11 runs? Suppose we want to fit a model with 11 different intercepts, for example. To do this we need to create 11 indicator variables. An **R** program to do this appears in Output 6.5.

---

[3] Available online at http://opr.princeton.edu/archive.

Output 6.5 Read the ELISA data and create indicators for each run number.

```
> data(DNase)
> ELISA <- DNase
> ELISA[1:5, ]                          # echo first few lines
    run   antigen optical
1     1 0.04882812   0.017
2     1 0.04882812   0.018
3     1 0.19531250   0.121
4     1 0.19531250   0.124
5     1 0.39062500   0.206
> (n <- dim(ELISA)[1])                   # number of rows
[1] 176
> runmax <- max(ELISA$run)               # number of runs
> ind <- matrix(0, n, runmax)            # initialize maxtrix of indicators
> for (j in 1:n) ind[ j , ELISA$run[j]] <- 1   # include 1's
> Ei <- cbind(ELISA, ind)                # append indicators to original data
> colnames(Ei)[4 : (3 + runmax)] <-      # create column names
+          gsub("100", "r", as.character(10001 : (10000 + runmax)))
> Ei[seq(1, n, 16),]                     # look at every 16-th
    run    antigen optical r01 r02 r03 r04 r05 r06 r07 r08 r09 r10 r11
1     1 0.04882812   0.017   1   0   0   0   0   0   0   0   0   0   0
17    2 0.04882812   0.045   0   1   0   0   0   0   0   0   0   0   0
33    3 0.04882812   0.070   0   0   1   0   0   0   0   0   0   0   0
49    4 0.04882812   0.011   0   0   0   1   0   0   0   0   0   0   0
65    5 0.04882812   0.035   0   0   0   0   1   0   0   0   0   0   0
81    6 0.04882812   0.086   0   0   0   0   0   1   0   0   0   0   0
97    7 0.04882812   0.094   0   0   0   0   0   0   1   0   0   0   0
113   8 0.04882812   0.054   0   0   0   0   0   0   0   1   0   0   0
129   9 0.04882812   0.032   0   0   0   0   0   0   0   0   1   0   0
145  10 0.04882812   0.052   0   0   0   0   0   0   0   0   0   1   0
161  11 0.04882812   0.047   0   0   0   0   0   0   0   0   0   0   1
```

The model statement can refer to all 11 indicators by writing

```
lm( optical ~ antigen + r02+r03+r04+r05+r06+r07+r08+r09+r10+r11,
        data = Ei)
```

and we leave out the indicator corresponding to the first run in order to avoid multico-linearity. This statement will fit a model with 11 separate intercepts, using the first run as the reference category.

Compare the output from this program to another where you include the log and square root of the antigen concentration. The difference may be because the relationship is not linear between the antigen concentration and resulting optical density.

Fit a model with 11 slopes. Create these as the interaction between the indicators for the run and the slope on antigen concentration.

7 Nonparametric Statistics

Do you remember all of the assumptions necessary in order for statistical inference to be valid when we perform a t-test? What happens if the variances aren't equal in the two groups? Do you need to test for this? What happens if the data is not normally distributed? How can you tell when it is? What happens if there are outliers? How do you know for sure whether a given data point is an outlier? While statisticians tend to be a cautious bunch, there is no need for you to be overly concerned. Nonparametric statistics are just the cure for messy data when outliers and highly skewed distributions would plague most analyses.

In a motivation for this chapter, suppose you learn the average salary at a company has increased but at the same time employees' median income is unchanged. This means most of the benefits were accrued by a few individuals, either at the top or at the bottom. In this example, is the average or the median more representative of the typical individual? We would like to cite a *robust* estimator, insensitive to a small number of unusually large or small values. In this example, we see the median remains unchanged if some of the largest or smallest values are altered.

> Nonparametric methods are used for continuous, but not necessarily normally distributed data, with possible outliers.

Nonparametric statistics are an entirely different approach to statistics. These include a wide variety of methods for the analysis of data with minimal assumptions about the underlying population. As an example, we might be able to rank different flavors of ice cream but would not be able to assign a quantitative value to those preferences.

7.1 A Test for Medians

Let us begin with an example from agriculture. Table 7.1 lists the dried weights of plants grown under either a control or a treated setting. The goal is to determine whether the treatment increases the dried plant weights.

Table 7.1 Dried weights of 20 plants grown under separate conditions.

Control:	4.17	5.58	5.18	6.11	4.50	4.61	5.17	4.53	5.33	5.14
Treated:	6.31	5.12	5.54	5.50	5.37	5.29	4.92	6.15	5.80	5.26

	Control	Treated
Means:	5.03	5.53
St. Dev.:	0.583	0.443

Source: Dobson (2002), Table 6.6, page 96.

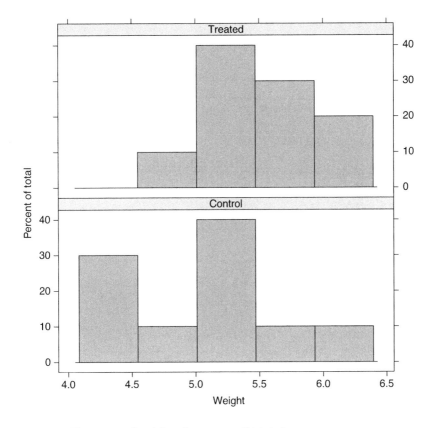

Figure 7.1 Histograms of weights of two types of dried plants.

The data in Table 7.1 is followed by group means and standard deviations. These summary values lead the reader to think of these data as two normal distributions. This may be far from the truth, of course. The paired histograms appear in Fig. 7.1. The relatively small sample sizes do not allow us to judge how normally distributed the data really is.

This figure was produced using the code in Output 7.1. The lattice package is a collection of graphical tools. You will have to install this package before you use it.

Output 7.1 Code to read plant, produce Fig. 7.1 and compare medians of two groups.

```
> plant <- read.table(file = "Plant Growth.txt", header = T, row.names = 1)
> plant[1:5,]                    # print the first five values to check
  weight group
1   4.17  ctrl
2   5.58  ctrl
3   5.18  ctrl
4   6.11  ctrl
5   4.50  ctrl
>
> require('lattice', 'RVAideMemoire') # be sure to install these packages
>
> histogram(~ weight | group, layout=c(1,2), data = plant)
>
> # Compare the medians of the plant values
>
> (med <- median(plant[ , 1]))        # pooled median
[1] 5.275
> mood.medtest(weight ~ group, data = plant)


Mood's median test

data:  weight by group
p-value = 0.1789


> (counts <- matrix(c(3,7,7,3), 2,2))    # perform our own chi-squared test
     [,1] [,2]
[1,]    3    7
[2,]    7    3
> chisq.test(counts)


Pearson's Chi-squared test with Yates' continuity correction

data:  counts
X-squared = 1.8, df = 1, p-value = 0.1797
```

From the pair of histograms in Fig. 7.1, we can see plants grown under the control conditions tend to be lighter and also have greater variability when compared with the treated plants. These conclusions are confirmed by looking at the means and standard deviations of the two groups.

One way to compare the two groups of plants is to compare their *medians*. Recall the median is the number evenly dividing the sample. Half of the observations are either above or below the median. In the present example, when we sort all 20 observations in the combined or *pooled* sample of both groups, we find the median of all

Table 7.2 The plant growth data summarized for the median test. The median is for the pooled sample.

	Control	Treated	Totals
> median	3	7	10
< median	7	3	10
Totals	10	10	20

observations falls between 5.26 and 5.29, both from the treated group. With an even number of observations, we average the two middle values, giving 5.275 as the pooled median. This value is found in Output 7.1 using the `median()` function in **R**.

Of all 20 observations in the pooled sample, we can see exactly half are above and half are below this value. If this median value of 5.275 is truly representative of the combined sample, then we would expect this statement will also be approximately true within each of the two groups of plants, as well. That is, about half of the controls and half of the treated plants should also be above or below this value. Let us see if this is the case.

Among the control plants, three had values above 5.275 and seven were below this value. Similarly, among the treated plants, seven were above 5.275 and three were below. We can summarize this finding in a 2×2 set of frequencies given in Table 7.2. Exercise 7.2 asks the reader to verify some properties of this table.

> The medians test examines the number of observations within each group above and below the pooled median.

We should immediately recognize the next step is to compute a Pearson chi-squared test on the data in Table 7.2. The value of the statistic is 3.2 (1 df) and p-value of 0.074. The presence of very small counts in this table suggests the chi-squared approximation might not be very accurate. The continuity-adjusted chi-square is 1.8 with $p = 0.18$, and the exact test also gives us $p = 0.18$, suggesting there is little difference in the weights of the two plant groups. (See Section 2.6 for a discussion of these different methods for examining the counts in a 2×2 table.) In the present case, the p-value of 0.18 seems more accurate.

It is also possible to skip the step of identifying the pooled median and the corresponding 2×2 table of counts with the **R** function

```
mood.medtest(weight ~ group, data = plant)
```

using syntax similar to what we use in `lm()`.

This function is illustrated in Output 7.1 and referred to as the Mood[1] test. The function is in the `RVAideMemoire` library.

---

[1] Alexander McFarlane Mood (1913–2009), US statistician.

Before we interpret the p-value for this table, we need to ask what is the hypothesis we are testing. The chi-squared statistic tests independence of rows and columns in this table, but how does independence relate to the problem of medians? The answer is if the rows are independent of the columns, then the distribution of the numbers of data points above and below the pooled median should be about the same for both groups of plants we are discussing. In other words, independence means the medians of separate plant groups should be close in value.

Suppose we went ahead and examined the usual Student t-test for this example. In such an examination of these data, we have $t = 2.13$ and $p = 0.048$. In words, the t-test provides strong evidence the treatment and control plants are different, but the medians test does not. Which approach is correct? Unfortunately, the answer is not so simple. If we are willing to assume the two populations of plants are normally distributed with the same variances, then the t-test is the correct way to proceed.

On the other hand, the medians test is very *robust* against misspecification of assumptions such as whether or not the data are normally distributed. The word *robust* is often used when describing a statistical procedure to mean it is insensitive to incorrect specifications or even gross outliers.

To convince ourselves of the robust properties of the medians test, suppose the value of the first treated plant was recorded as 7.31 rather than as 6.31. Such errors are more common than you might expect. If this were the case, then the frequencies in Table 7.2 would remain unchanged. Some might argue the value of 7.31 is still a valid data point. Suppose the value was recorded as 63.1 rather than 6.31. In this case, the median test would again remain unchanged, but this extreme value would have a great effect on the t-test. The t-test would reject the null hypothesis of no treatment difference.

The point here is some outliers might not be recognized as such and could produce misleading results. Of course, if there are no outliers, we pay a price for our caution. As we see in this example, the medians test is unable to detect an alternative hypothesis the t-test finds statistically significant. Notice also the t-test compares the two means, but the medians test compares the medians. In symmetric distributions, such as the normal, these two measures will coincide. If the data is skewed, then these may be very different.

> Nonparametric methods are insensitive to model assumptions
> and outliers but have reduced power.

So, in conclusion, are the treated plants heavier than the control plants? In this example there do not appear to be large departures from the assumptions of equal variances and normally distributed data, so the t-test seems appropriate. Inference based on the t-test indicates the treated plants are heavier, and this appears to be a reasonable conclusion. Perhaps our use of the medians test was overly cautious. There is no telling what might happen the next time we are faced with a similar situation, of course. The medians test is a good tool to remember for situations when the data do not conform to the assumptions as well as in this example.

In a critical situation when the statistical significance is very important to us, the only fair approach is to specify the statistical analysis before we are able to observe the data. Otherwise we might be accused of fishing for the statistical method achieving the most extreme level of significance, hence distorting its interpretation. Although such a level of caution is unnecessary in the present example involving plant weights, there are times when an honest and unbiased assessment of statistical significance is essential. Such an example might include a clinical trial of a new experimental drug in which we need an accurate measure of its efficacy.

This plant data example is continued in Exercise 7.8. There were two treatment groups in addition to the control group of plants. Simultaneous comparisons of more than two groups can be done in the mood.test procedure. This is illustrated in Exercise 7.8.

7.2   Elementary School Math Achievement Scores

Elementary school education is constantly being evaluated and new teaching methods are being introduced. Progress is measured by standardized tests given by the schools to the children. The tests are designed to identify poor or failing schools but also point out successful programs. Among many criticisms of the program are claims teachers are coaching their students in test-taking skills rather than covering subject-matter material and critical thinking. Nevertheless, schools systems with improving records are quick to publicize their results. One summary from New York State Department of Education appears in Fig. 7.2, comparing mathematics test scores in elementaty schools for the years 2018 and 2019.

Without exception, in every possible category of age and race, in both the city and the state, there was an improvement. How is it possible every grade in both New York City and State and every racial/ethnic group shows an improvement in math scores? Can we assign a p-value to this outcome? The null hypothesis is nothing has changed in teaching methods and the test scores should be about the same between the two years.

We could use a Student t-test to compare differences in the two years' results, but the figure is missing the numerical values of both the means and standard deviations. Instead, we can simply use the increase or decrease as a binary-valued outcome, regardless of the actual amount of change. If each year's test scores are comparable to the previous year's, then it should be equally likely to rise or fall.

Consider tossing a coin six times, corresponding to whether there was an improvement in each of the state-wide grades 3 through 8. What is the probability of observing six heads in six tosses of a fair coin? The answer is

$$\frac{1}{2^6} = \frac{1}{64} = 0.015625.$$

Perhaps we should consider a two-tailed test for this outcome. That would have us ask the question, "What are the chances the change is in the same direction for all

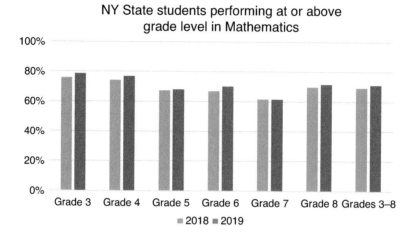

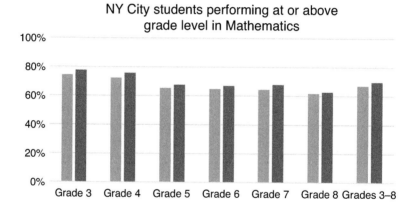

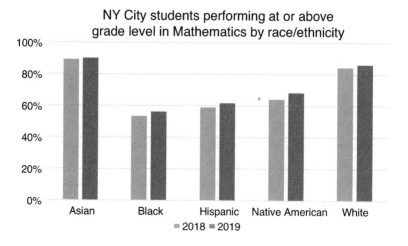

Figure 7.2 Math achievement scores among elementary school students.
Source: New York State Education Department.

grades 3 through 8?". In terms of nonparametric statistics, this is also expressible as the probability of either six heads or six tails in six tosses of a fair coin. In this case, the probability is 0.03125. In either the one- or two-tailed test, these probabilities are still small. If we included the data from New York City then there would be twice as many coin tosses resulting in the same outcome, yielding a much more remarkable p-value.

The fifth graders in 2018 became the sixth graders in 2019, so maybe the analogy to coin tosses is not quite independent. Also, test scores improved in both the city and also in the state. These outcomes are also not independent, because the city is included as part of the state. The improvement in scores appears across all ethnic/racial groups, and these are also included in the city and state data.

How can we explain this finding? Did large numbers of underachievers drop out each year, resulting in better scores year after year? Are the tests comparable in different years? We appear to reject the hypothesis that the 2018 and 2019 tests are comparable in favor of some other explanation. Maybe teachers and teaching methods suddenly became much better. We cannot claim the students suddenly became smarter, because they appear more than once in this table.

Standardized tests such as the GRE and the SAT are said to be *equated* by the administrators so the results can be compared from one year to the next. Was this done with the test values summarized in this figure? There are conferences among educators and statisticians discussing how and whether equating should be done.

The nonparametric analysis of these data reduces the year-to-year comparison of math scores to the results of a simple coin toss. The actual magnitudes of the differences might be compared using a t-test. Instead, in this nonparametric statistical analysis, we are only looking at the *direction* of change, not the actual amount.

7.3   Rank Sum Test

The medians test and the examination of the math test scores in Section 7.2 reduce every observation to a coin toss. Specifically, the medians test judges every observation as being either above or below the pooled sample median. The actual magnitude of every observation is lost. It does not matter how far above or below the median an observation is. Does this seem like a tremendous loss of information? Rank methods meet this loss halfway: Instead of reducing all observations to binary above/below status, rank methods replace the actual observations with their ordered value when the data is sorted.

To illustrate this method, consider again the plant growth data from Table 7.1. All 20 of the pooled sample values are sorted in Table 7.3 from smallest to largest and identified as belonging to either the control or the treated groups. Each observation is also identified with its rank or order number, from 1 to 20 in terms of the pooled sample. So, for example, the four smallest observations (ranked 1 to 4) are associated with the control group, and then the next two smallest observations (ranked 5 and 6) are in the treated group.

Table 7.3 The plant growth data from Table 7.1 converted to ranks.

Control	4.17	4.50	4.53	4.61			5.14	5.17	5.18	
Treated					4.92	5.12				5.26
Rank	1	2	3	4	5	6	7	8	9	10

Control		5.33				5.58		6.11		
Treated	5.29		5.37	5.50	5.54		5.80		6.15	6.31
Rank	11	12	13	14	15	16	17	18	19	20

Output 7.2 Program to compare the two groups of plants in Table 7.1.

```
> wilcox.test(weight ~ group,  data = plant)

Wilcoxon rank sum test

data:  weight by group
W = 25, p-value = 0.06301
alternative hypothesis: true location shift is not equal to 0
```

> In rank statistical methods, the original observations are replaced
> by their ranks when the values are sorted.

In rank methods, we replace the observations by their ranks. A large observation achieves a high rank, unlike the medians test where all observations larger than the median are treated equally. In Table 7.3, if both the treated and the control plants had roughly the same means, then we would also expect these two samples to have roughly the same average rank values. In Output 7.2, the Wilcoxon[2] test is used to compare the ranks.

The sum of ranks for the control plants is 80 and for the treated plants it is 130. If the two groups of plants had the same distribution, then these values should be close together. The actual distribution of the sum of the ranks is developed in the theory behind the Wilcoxon test but is not needed for us to appreciate the use of the method.

The statistical significance of the rank sum test is 0.063 in this example. Compare this to the p-value of 0.18 obtained using the median test, demonstrating the increase in power over the median test illustrated in Output 7.1. There are one- and two-tailed versions of the rank sum test, just as in the Student t-test. In Exercise 7.8, a third group of plants is introduced and compared with the others.

---

[2] Frank Wilcoxon (1892–1965), US statistician and chemist.

Table 7.4 Health statistics on the 50 states and District of Columbia.

	Physicians	Vaccination rate	Prenatal care	Low birth weight	Mortality Age adjusted	Neonatal
Alabama	21.4	79	82.8	10.35	1004.0	5.4
Alaska	24.1	67	80.0	6.02	781.5	2.9
Arizona	22.5	71	76.4	7.05	775.2	4.3
Arkansas	20.4	73	79.5	9.04	934.6	5.2
			· · · ·			
West Virginia	25.2	68	85.8	9.16	974.1	4.9
Wisconsin	25.7	81	84.0	6.93	758.3	4.4
Wyoming	19.4	64	82.9	8.71	814.6	4.6
United States	26.9	77%	83.2%	8.07	812.0	4.6

Source: Centers for Disease Control.

7.4 Ranking and the Healthiest State

Do you feel comfortable with ranked data rather than the actual values? We have all seen rankings of the "best" cities to live in and the "best" colleges to attend. There are popular websites ranking the best (and worst) dressed celebrities. There is even a ranking of the New York City subway lines.[3] The actual ranking depends on how much weight we give to each of the criteria going into the ranking.

As an example of how such a ranking might be conducted, let us take some public health data[4] collected on each of the 50 states and the District of Columbia given in Table 7.4. For each state, we have the number of physicians per 10,000 population, the rate of childhood vaccination, the rate of prenatal care, the rate of low-birth-weight infants, and infant and age-adjusted mortality.

Let us see how we might rank the different states on their degree of health. This requires us to construct a scale of health. This scale is rather arbitrary and depends on which criteria we value most. As an example, we might say health depends on low infant mortality and high childhood vaccination rates. This first health measure is then defined as

$$\text{Health}_1 = \text{vaccine rate} - 10 \times \text{infant mortality}$$

ignoring all other information available.

Notice infant mortality rate is given a negative weight because large values are unhealthy. The multiple of 10 in this weighting is also arbitrary. The healthiest state using this criterion is Massachusetts, with a score of 47. Iowa and Minnesota are both tied for second place with scores of 45. The District of Columbia is worst.

---

[3] Really. See www.straphangers.org/reports/StateoftheSubways2016.pdf.
[4] Available online at www.cdc.gov/nchs/data/hus/hus07.pdf.

For another example of ranking, suppose we decide a low overall mortality rate and a large number of physicians is more important. Then we might decide on the second health measure

$$\text{Health}_2 = 100 \times \text{Physicians} - \text{mortality}.$$

If we use this metric then Washington, DC, is the healthiest, largely because of a very large number of physicians living in the city. In other words, Washington, DC, is either ranked as the most healthy or the worst, depending on the criteria we use.

Watch for similar rankings reported in the popular press, and be ready to ask for details about the methodology used to create the rankings. The data from this section is examined in Exercise 7.11. Consider developing a method making your state the healthiest.

7.5   Nonparametric Regression: LOESS

There are also nonparametric regression methods. Suppose we want to show how the values of an outcome variable y are related to an explanatory variable x, but we are not sure if a straight-line relationship is appropriate. Maybe the best descriptive relationship is a straight-line, or maybe a polynomial. Maybe some transformation of either x or y might be better. This is the spirit of nonparametric statistics: We don't want to make any more assumptions than necessary.

Suppose, however, we are willing to say the relationship between the mean value of y and x is smooth. A small change in x should not greatly change the mean of y. We cannot commit ourselves to much more than this statement. LOESS (pronounced and sometimes also written as LOWESS) is the abbreviation for locally weighted scatter-plot smoothing. Very simply, LOESS represents a compromise between minimizing the sum of squared residuals and providing a smooth response model.

Too much roughness may produce a smaller sum of squared errors. But a model with many wiggles is not a simple summary of the data. At the other extreme, the ultimate smooth fit says the best description of the y values is their mean. This flat-line model is usually not of much use to us either, and we should be able to do better.

Let us consider fitting a LOESS model to the gasoline consumption data examined in Section 6.4. We showed taking logs of the per-person consumption of gasoline was much better than examining the original consumption values. Figure 7.3 displays a smooth fit and its corresponding 95% confidence interval. The **R** program fitting the LOESS curve to these data is given in Output 7.3. In this code for `loess` we chose an optimal smoothing parameter (`span = 1`) making a compromise between a good fit and a smooth model.

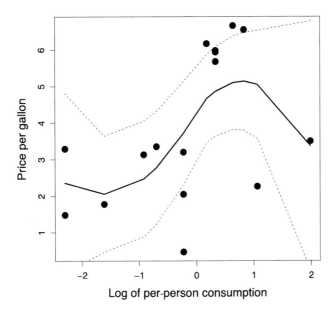

Figure 7.3 LOESS fit and its 95% confidence interval for the gasoline consumption data.

Output 7.3 Program to fit and plot the LOESS curve to the gasoline consumption data in Fig. 7.3.

```
gas <- read.table(file = "gasoline.txt", header = T)
gas[1:3, ]                              # print a few lines
lcon <- log(gas$consume)                # log consumption
ol <- order(lcon)                       # ordering of values
lcon <- lcon[ol]                        # sorted log consumption
ppg <- gas$price[ol]                    # corresponding ordered prices

plot(ppg ~ lcon, ylab = "Price per gallon",    # plot the original data
     xlab = "Log of per person consumption", pch = 19,
     cex = 1.75, cex.lab = 1.5)
lo <- loess(ppg ~ lcon, span = 1)       # create the LOESS object
prd <- predict(lo, se=T)                # summary statistics
lines(lcon, prd$fit, lwd = 2.5)         # add fitted LOESS to plot
                                        # add 95% confidence interval
lines(lcon, prd$fit - qt(0.975, prd$df) * prd$se, lty=2)
lines(lcon, prd$fit + qt(0.975, prd$df) * prd$se, lty=2)
```

The center curve in Fig. 7.3 is the LOESS fit, and the outer two represent the 95% confidence interval of the LOESS fit. We can see the price of gasoline is relatively flat for the lower half of the consumption values, but jumps up corresponding to the higher consuming northern European nations. The highest consumption and relatively

---

Output 7.4 Program to plot three LOESS curves in Fig. 7.4.

```
gas <- read.table(file = "gasoline.txt", header = T)
gas[1:3, ]
lcon <- log(gas$consume)
scatter.smooth(lcon, gas$price, span = .4, ylab = "Price per gallon",
          xlab = "Log of per person consumption",
          pch = 19, cex = 1.75, cex.lab = 1.5)
lines(loess.smooth(lcon, gas$price, span = .7), lwd = 2)
lines(loess.smooth(lcon, gas$price, span = 1), lwd = 4)  # smoothest
```

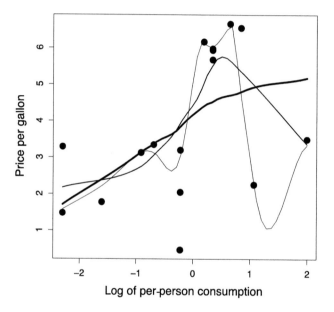

Figure 7.4 Three LOESS smoothing fits for the gasoline data. Darker lines are smoother models.

low prices in the United States and Singapore cause the LOESS fit to fall again at the right side of this figure.

Perhaps we may still feel the low prices in the United States and Singapore provide too much leverage and the fitted model is not quite smooth enough. It is possible to adjust the LOESS smoothing parameter to determine the compromise between smoothness and good fit. The code in Output 7.4 provides three smoothing parameters as values to the span. Larger values of span are smoother and lower values will have a better fit. A reasonable range to consider is between 0.5 and 1.5 in most cases.

These three different smoothing parameters produce the models given in Fig. 7.4. Smoother models are plotted using darker lines. A smoothing parameter of 0.4 produces a model with several small twists and turns, trying to follow the observed data too closely. A value of 0.7 produces a much smoother fit, but the model is still trying to drop in order to accommodate the data values from the United States and Singapore. The smoothest graph uses a smoothing value of 1. This model shows price is fairly flat across nations with the lowest gasoline consumption, rises in the middle, and then levels off again. In this example, the smoothest of the three LOESS models seems to provide the best summary of the data on the basis of this simple summary.

7.6 Exercises

7.1 What are the assumptions of a t-test?

7.2 Why are the row and column sums all equal to 10 in Table 7.2? In this medians test, would the results be any different if we took logs of the weight data? Would the results change if we took logs before performing the t-test or the rank sum test? Why? If you can't answer these questions right away, try it with some data and see what happens.

7.3 Verify sums of ranks in Table 7.3 are 80 for the controls and 130 for the treated plants. Verify the sum of all ranks available in 20 observations is equal to

$$1 + 2 + \cdots + 20 = 210.$$

Hint: Write this sum as

$$(1 + 20) + (2 + 19) + \cdots + (10 + 11).$$

7.4 Which of the smooth fitted models of Fig. 7.4 do you prefer: the best-fitting model or the smoothest fit? The smoothest fit also provides a relatively simple description for the data. This is an important goal in statistics.

7.5 The diastolic blood pressures of subjects who were treated and of untreated controls are listed here.

> **Treated:** 92 108 112 90 88
> **Controls:** 83 90 78 90 90 106 92 78 103 98

Compare these two groups using nonparametric methods and the t-test. Do you have more confidence in one or the other of these two methods? Are there any data values you feel might provide too much influence on the t-test? Try changing one of the data values to see how much this varies the conclusions of the two different statistical methods. What does this say about how robust these different methods are?

7.6 Reexamine the fusion time data in Table 2.1. Use both the medians and the rank sum tests to see if there is a statistically significant difference between these two groups. Do the significance levels you find agree with those using a t-test? Suppose we multiply some of the largest observed values by some large number. Does this change our statistical inference based on the t-test? Are the medians and rank sum tests changed by this action?

Table 7.5 The full data on plant weights.

Control:	4.17	5.58	5.18	6.11	4.50	4.61	5.17	4.53	5.33	5.14
Treatment 1:	4.81	4.17	4.41	3.59	5.87	3.83	6.03	4.89	4.32	4.69
Treatment 2:	6.31	5.12	5.54	5.50	5.37	5.29	4.92	6.15	5.80	5.26

7.7 In pharmacokinetics, we often want to know how long it takes for a drug to reach its peak serum concentration. This time is called T_{max}. The subject's blood is not sampled continuously, but rather at irregular time points following the administration of the drug. Here are the results of T_{max} for an experiment comparing two different formulations of a pain reliever, rounded to the nearest quarter of an hour.

> **Standard formulation:** 1.0 1.25 1.5 1.5 1.0 1.25 1.0 1.5
> **New formulation:** 0.5 0.75 0.5 1.0 0.75 1.25 1.0 1.5

Compare the T_{max} values for these two formulations using the t-test, the median test and the rank method. Which of these methods do you feel provides a more reliable conclusion? Explain why.

7.8 The plant growth data in Table 7.1 is part of a larger experiment involving two treatments in addition to a control group of plants. The full data set is given in Table 7.5. Each of the three groups of experimental conditions contained 10 plants. This exercise asks you to develop a generalization of the medians test described in Section 7.1 to test for simultaneous differences between the medians of these three groups.

Begin by finding the median of the sample pooled over all three groups. Within each of the three groups, count the numbers of observations above and below this pooled median. Express these frequencies in a 2 × 3 table of counts and then compute the usual 2 df Pearson chi-squared statistic on this table testing for independence of rows and columns. Does this agree with the result from the mood.test? Express the null and alternative hypotheses for this test in terms of the comparisons of the medians.

7.9 Reexamine the Swiss fertility data in Table 6.9. Consider the relationship between fertility rates and the percentage of population with higher education levels. Use LOESS to show the smooth, nonparametric relationship between fertility and education is nearly a straight line.

In the exercise of Section 6.6.7, we suggested taking logs of education in order to remove the influence of the few highly educated provinces. Use LOESS to model fertility in terms of log education. Notice the smooth fit on log education has a very different form. Interpret this model in simple, nonmathematical terms.

7.10 A group of mentally deficient children were enrolled in a speech therapy program. These children were classified as either aphasic or mentally retarded. Their scores on the Vineland Social Maturity Scale were as follows.

Aphasic: 56 43 30 97 67 24 76 49 46 29 46 83 93 38 25 44 66 71 54 20 25

Mentally Retarded: 90 53 32 44 47 42 58 16 49 54 81 59 35 81 41 24 41 61 31 20

How do these two groups differ? Compare these two groups using a t-test and nonparametric methods. Plot the data using boxplots and with a jittered group to see if the values appear to be sampled from a normal distribution. (Data source: Glovsky and Rigrodsky, 1964.)

7.11 Examine the data in Table 7.4 and provide your own ranking of the healthiest state. Can you provide an intuitive reason for your ranking method?

7.6.1   Cloth Run-Up

The data in Table 7.6 represents the percentage of cloth run-up (wasted) by each of five different suppliers to a clothing manufacturer.[5] The values in this table are

Table 7.6 Cloth run-up from five suppliers.

	Supplier			
A	B	C	D	E
1.2	16.4	12.1	11.5	24.0
10.1	−6.0	9.7	10.2	−3.7
−2.0	−11.6	7.4	3.8	8.2
1.5	−1.3	−2.1	8.3	9.2
−3.0	4.0	10.1	6.6	−9.3
−0.7	17.0	4.7	10.2	8.0
3.2	3.8	4.6	8.8	15.8
2.7	4.3	3.9	2.7	22.3
−3.2	10.4	3.6	5.1	3.1
−1.7	4.2	9.6	11.2	16.8
2.4	8.5	9.8	5.9	11.3
0.3	6.3	6.5	13.0	12.3
3.5	9.0	5.7	6.8	16.9
−0.8	7.1	5.1	14.5	
19.4	4.3	3.4	5.2	
2.8	19.7	−0.8	7.3	
13.0	3.0	−3.9	7.1	
42.7	7.6	0.9	3.4	
1.4	70.2	1.5	0.7	
3.0	8.5			
2.4	6.0			
1.3	2.9			

[5] Data and other analyses available at www.coursehero.com/file/p1ah31kd/Test-at-the-1-level-Table-1133-Run-ups-for-Different-Plants-Making-Levi-Strauss/.

comparisons to the manufacturer's computer model suggesting how much cloth will be run-up. A negative number is possible if the supplier is careful and manages to lose less material than anticipated by this model.

Examine a boxplot for percentage run-up by each of the five suppliers. Is there evidence all five have the same variability? (See Exercise 6.5 for an examination of the assumptions of a one-way ANOVA.) Is a one-way ANOVA an appropriate way to compare the five suppliers? Is this method affected by the exclusion of any outliers you see?

Does a nonparametric approach reach a different conclusion? Are the five suppliers about the same or are there real differences? Can you identify good or bad ones? Which is a better property: consistency (i.e., a small variance) or low mean run-up?

7.6.2   Prices of Beanie Babies

Beanie Babies are small cloth toys filled with plastic beads. Collecting and investing in these was a popular fad in the 1990s. These animal models come in a wide variety of colors, and small variations can result in large differences in their value to collectors. The prices (as of the year 2000) and year of production (often referred to as "birth date") are given in Table 7.7. Also included is an indicator of whether the item is currently being manufactured or retired. The price is often determined by what collectors are willing to pay. As a result, there are some extreme outliers here. Be sure to identify these.

Compare the prices for current and retired items. Begin by examining the means and standard deviations in **R**. Plot the data. Does jittering the current/retired status indicator help you see the distribution of values?

Perform a t-test. Do you have confidence in the assumptions for this method? What do you learn using the median or rank sum tests? Do the nonparametric methods seem more appropriate? Explain why.

Table 7.7 Value of Beanie Babies with production year and whether current (0) or retired (1).

Name	$ Value	Retired?	Year
Ally, Alligator	30.00	1	1994
Almond, Beige Bear	11.00	0	1999
Amber, Gold Tabby	10.00	0	1998
Ants, Anteater	10.00	1	1997
. . . . . .			
Zero, Penguin	14.00	1	1998
Ziggy, Zebra	15.00	1	1995
Zip, Black Cat, pink ears, no white paws	900.00	1	1994
Zip, Black Cat, white face/belly	350.00	1	1994
Zip, Black Cat, newly retired	30.00	1	1994

Table 7.8 Subject outcomes and the four cracker diets.

Cracker type	Diet	Subject no.	Calories digested	Bloat?	Cracker type	Diet	Subject no.	Calories digested	Bloat?
control	1	3	1772.84	none	bran	4	3	1752.63	low
combo	3	9	2121.97	med	gum	2	4	2558.61	high
gum	2	1	2026.91	med	bran	4	1	2047.42	low
⋮									
gum	2	12	2166.77	med	bran	4	12	2287.52	none

A vailable at `https://dasl.datadescription.com/datafile/diet/`.

How would you use the production year in a linear regression? Should the slope be positive or negative if older models are more valuable? Is it? Try LOESS and see if you can make a simple statement about the relationship between age and price.

7.6.3   The Cracker Diet

A cracker manufacturer thought it would make for good marketing if they could advertise their product as a way to lose weight. An experiment was conducted to see if eating their crackers before a meal would reduce hunger and decrease the urge to consume a higher number of calories. Twelve overweight women were recruited and asked to eat one of four different fiber crackers: a control with no additive; gum added; bran added; or a combination of bran and gum. They were allowed to eat as much as they wanted in a monitored meal. The number of calories they consumed was carefully measured.

An unfortunate side effect of the diet was feelings of gastric upset or bloating reported by many of the subjects. The results from this experiment, including the number of calories consumed, are given in Table 7.8. Subjects were examined once for each of the four different cracker types. In this exercise let us assume these multiple measurements on the same person are independent of each other.

Is the feeling of bloat related to the diet? Summarize the data in a 4 × 4 table of frequencies using the different row and column categories of diet and bloating. Perform a chi-squared test to see if these are independent of each other. The exact test of significance may be a better choice than the chi-squared test because of the small counts in this table. You might review the discussion of these methods given in Section 2.6.

In each of the 16 categories, compare the observed and expected counts. Are some of the diets more likely to result in bloating? Can you make a convincing case for this? Consider combining rows and columns in this table to make your argument clearer.

Is there a difference between the four diets with regard to the number of calories consumed? Does a boxplot reveal any outliers? Run `npar1way` and examine the differences using indicator variables in a regression as well as a nonparametric method. Which of these methods seems appropriate to make the comparison? Do these methods come to the same or different conclusions when comparing the four diets?

8   Logistic Regression

Everything we have discussed so far has been concerned with models for the means of normally or, at the least, continuously distributed data. The rest of this book is about models for other distributions. This chapter discusses models for data sampled from a binomial distribution. Logistic regression is the preferred method for examining this type of data. These methods are different from what we have seen so far. At the same time, you will recognize a lot of similar features.

8.1   Example: an Insecticide Experiment

Let's begin with an example of the type of data lending itself to this analysis. Consider the experimental data summarized in Table 8.1. There were six large jars, each containing a number of beetles and a carefully measured, small amount of insecticide. After a specified amount of time, the experimenters examined the number of beetles still alive. We can calculate the empirical death rate for each jar's level of exposure to the insecticide. These are given in the last row of Table 8.1 using

$$\text{Mortality rate} = \frac{\text{Number died}}{\text{Number exposed}}.$$

How can we develop statistical models to describe this data? We should immediately recognize the outcomes within each jar are binary valued: alive or dead. We can probably assume these events are independent of each other. The counts of alive or dead should then follow the binomial distribution. (See Section 2.1 for a quick review of this important statistical model.)

There are six separate and independent binomial experiments in this example. The N parameters for the binomial models are the number of insects in each jar. Similarly, the p parameters represent the mortality probabilities in each jar. The aim is to model the p parameters of these six binomial experiments. Any models we develop for this data will need to incorporate something about the various insecticide dose levels to describe the mortality probability p in each jar. The alert reader will notice the empirical mortality rates given in the last row of Table 8.1 are not monotonically

Table 8.1 Mortality of beetles exposed to various doses of an insecticide.

Dead	15	24	26	24	29	29
Alive	35	25	24	26	21	20
Number exposed	50	49	50	50	50	49
Exposure dose	1.082	1.161	1.212	1.258	1.310	1.348
Mortality rate	0.30	0.49	0.52	0.48	0.58	0.59

Source: Plackett (1981).

increasing with increasing exposure levels of the insecticide. Despite this remark, there is no reason for us to fit a nonmonotonic model to these data.

> Use logistic regression to model the p parameter in data
> sampled from a binomial distribution.

The aim of this chapter is to explain models for the different values of the p parameters using the values of the doses of the insecticide in each jar. The first approach might be to treat the outcomes as normally distributed. All of the ns are large, so a normal approximation to the binomial distributions should work. We also already know a lot about linear regression, so we are tempted to fit the linear model

$$p = \beta_0 + \beta_1 \text{Dose} + \text{error} .$$

What is wrong with this approach? It seems simple enough, but remember the p must always be between 0 and 1. There is no guarantee at extreme values of the Dose, this straight-line model would result in estimates of p less than 0 or greater than 1. We would expect a good model for these data to always give an estimate of p between 0 and 1. A second but less striking problem is the variance of the binomial distribution is not the same for different values of the p parameter. The assumption of constant variance is not valid for the usual linear regression.

8.2   The Logit Transformation

We like the idea of fitting straight lines but have not yet encountered a constraint on the fitted model, such as p always remaining between 0 and 1, as in this case. The solution is to introduce a new class of models. We define the *logit* of p as the logarithm (base e) of the odds. Mathematically,

$$\text{logit}(p) = \log \frac{p}{1 - p} . \tag{8.1}$$

The ratio $p/(1 - p)$ is the odds, or ratio of the probability of the event (in this case, insect death) to the probability of the complementary event (again, in this case, a living insect). The *odds ratio* is familiar to epidemiologists and horse-race handicappers alike. The logit is the log-odds of an event occurring. In epidemiology, we usually talk about the odds rather than the probability of an event, especially when the events are rare.

It does not matter much which event is considered a success or failure in the binomial distribution. Recall the property of the logarithm of a reciprocal: For any positive number z

$$\log(1/z) = -\log(z)$$

so we have

$$\text{logit}(p) = \log \frac{p}{1-p} = -\log \frac{1-p}{p} = -\text{logit}(1-p). \qquad (8.2)$$

That is, the logit of success is the negative of the logit of failure. We only need to remember which outcome we are calling a success.

> The logit is the log-odds of the probability.

Let us take a moment to motivate the use of the logit. The p parameter is restricted to values between 0 and 1. The logit transforms p to cover the entire number line. A plot of $\text{logit}(p)$ against p is given in Fig. 8.1. From this figure, we see how values

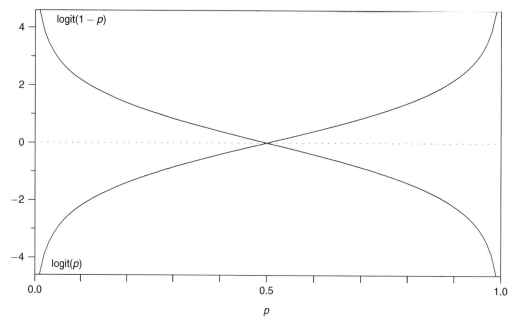

Figure 8.1 Plot of $\text{logit}(p)$ and $\text{logit}(1-p)$ against p.

of p are spread out from the interval of 0 to 1 onto the entire number line. As p gets very close to 0 or 1, this transformation takes on extremely large negative and positive values, respectively.

From this figure we can see logit(p) is 0 when p is 1/2. Similarly, logit(p) is positive for p greater than 1/2, and logit(p) is negative when p is less than 1/2. The plot of logit($1 - p$) in this figure demonstrates the relation given in (8.2), namely, the logit of failure is the negative of the logit of success.

Logistic regression is the statistical method in which we model the logit(p) in terms of the explanatory variables available to us. In the specific case of the beetle data in Table 8.1, we have

$$\text{logit}(p) = \beta_0 + \beta_1 \text{Dose}, \tag{8.3}$$

where the intercept and slope parameters β_0 and β_1 are estimated in **R**.

On the right-hand side of this relationship, we see the familiar linear summary of the explanatory variable we encountered in linear regression in Chapter 3. The logit on the left side of this model is the nonlinear transformed value of the binomial p parameter.

> Logistic regression specifies the logit of p is a linear
> combination of the risk factors.

The relationship in (8.3) can be solved for p in terms of the Dose, giving us

$$p = \frac{\exp\{\beta_0 + \beta_1 \text{Dose}\}}{1 + \exp\{\beta_0 + \beta_1 \text{Dose}\}}. \tag{8.4}$$

The exponential function ($\exp(z) = e^z$) is always positive, and the denominator is always 1 more than the numerator. This shows the model produces values of p between 0 and 1 regardless of the values of the parameters β_0, β_1, and the Dose of the insecticide. The relationships in (8.3) and (8.4) are equivalent. These two different forms both appear in published literature using logistic regression.

Let us end this section with a description of another method closely allied with logistic regression. The relation in (8.3) is not the only method used to model p in linear terms of the insecticide dose while maintaining the restriction of p between 0 and 1.

Another popular method used to model the p parameter for binomial data is called the *probit* model. The probit of p is related to the area under the normal curve.

More specifically, *probit regression* is the area under the normal curve to the left of

$$\alpha_0 + \alpha_1 \text{ Dose},$$

where the intercept α_0 and slope α_1 are parameters estimated in **R**. All normal areas are positive and less than 1, so we are assured all values of p will always be between 0 and 1.

The parameters β_0 and β_1 of the fitted logistic model and α_0 and α_1 of the fitted probit model will be different but will generally exhibit similar statistical significance levels. The interpretations of the logit and probit models are very different but, as we demonstrate in Fig. 8.2 in Section 8.3, the fitted models are usually in close agreement. The reason for this agreement is not obvious, but we might think of the logistic model as a t-distribution with a small number of degrees of freedom, while the probit follows a normal shape. In Fig. 2.6 we see these are not very different from the normal distribution.

We use the term *link* to describe the connection of the p parameter and the linear function of the Dose. We have just described two link functions for these data: the logistic link and the probit link. There are other link functions available for binary-valued data in **R**. These include the complementary log–log link.

8.3   Logistic Regression in R

The program to fit a logistic model to the beetle data is given in Output 8.1. There are also many regression diagnostics produced by the program, similar to those developed for linear regression. These diagnostics are discussed in Chapter 9. Right now we want to emphasize the computing and interpretation of the models.

In Output 8.1 we begin by reading the data. Get in to the habit of printing out enough of the data to convince yourself this was done correctly. The vector of paired responses, denoted `resp`, consists of two columns: the number of bugs dead and alive, respectively. The `cbind` function joins two or more columns of data.

The `glm` program for generalized linear models has a syntax similar to the `lm` program but allows you to specify the distribution of the response values, in this case binomial, as well as a choice of link. The `glm` regression program also produces residuals and regression diagnostics, explained in the following chapter.

After the $\sim$ sign in `glm`, we can list any number of explanatory variables we want to put into the model. The program will fit a slope for each variable and an intercept. These appear in the abbreviated Output 8.2. Both the slope and intercept are presented as estimated values, standard errors, and tests of statistical significance, very similar to the output from `lm` for normally distributed data. In Output 8.2 we see strong evidence the slope on `dose` is nonzero. If we judged this slope to be zero (i.e., the null hypothesis) then we infer there is no relationship between dose of exposure and mortality.

Part of the output from the program in Output 8.1 is given in Output 8.2. There is much more output than this, and it is explained in Chapter 9. Output 8.2 includes a portion very similar to what we saw in the output for linear regression. Specifically, there are parameter estimates, estimated standard errors for these, tests of statistical significance, and a confidence interval for the slope. Let us go over these before we proceed.

Output 8.1 **R** program to fit logistic regression models for the pesticide experiment in Table 8.1.

```
> bugs <- read.table(file = "beetle.txt", header = TRUE)
> bugs                          # echo the data
  died  N  dose
1   15 50 1.082
2   24 49 1.161
3   26 50 1.212
4   24 50 1.258
5   29 50 1.310
6   29 49 1.348
> lived <- N - died
> resp <- cbind(died, lived)  # create response values
> resp                         # check response values
      died lived
[1,]   15    35
[2,]   24    25
[3,]   26    24
[4,]   24    26
[5,]   29    21
[6,]   29    20
> glm(resp ~ dose, family = binomial)     # logit is the default link

Call:  glm(formula = resp ~ dose, family = binomial)

Coefficients:
(Intercept)        dose
     -4.898       3.964


      .   .   .


> glm(resp ~ dose, family = binomial(link = probit)) # fit probit

Call:  glm(formula = resp ~ dose, family = binomial(link = probit))

Coefficients:
(Intercept)        dose
     -3.064       2.479


      .   .   .
```

Output 8.2 Analysis of logistic parameter estimates from Output 8.1.

```
> logit.out <- glm(resp ~ dose, family = binomial)
> summary(logit.out)
```

. . .

```
Coefficients:
            Estimate Std. Error z value Pr(>|z|)
(Intercept)   -4.898      1.645  -2.977  0.00291 **
dose           3.964      1.335   2.970  0.00298 **
---
Signif. codes:  0 '***' 0.001 '**' 0.01 '*' 0.05 '.' 0.1 ' ' 1
```

. . .

Output 8.3 Analysis of parameter estimates of probit regression.

```
> probit.out <- glm(resp ~ dose, family = binomial(link = probit))
> summary(probit.out)
```

. . . . .

```
Coefficients:
            Estimate Std. Error z value Pr(>|z|)
(Intercept)  -3.0636     1.0175  -3.011  0.00261 **
dose          2.4794     0.8258   3.002  0.00268 **
---
Signif. codes:  0 '***' 0.001 '**' 0.01 '*' 0.05 '.' 0.1 ' ' 1
```

. . . . . .

The fitted logistic regression model in Output 8.2 is

$$\text{logit}(\hat{p}) = -4.898 + 3.964\,\text{Dose} \tag{8.5}$$

or equivalently

$$\hat{p} = \frac{\exp(-4.898 + 3.964\,\text{Dose})}{1 + \exp(-4.898 + 3.964\,\text{Dose})}.$$

This fitted logistic function of Dose is plotted in Fig. 8.2.

Both the intercept and slope have estimated standard errors given in Output 8.2. The z-value statistic is

$$z = \frac{\text{parameter estimate}}{\text{standard error}},$$

and behaves as a standard normal under the null hypothesis: The underlying parameter being estimated is equal to 0.

The p-value associated with this test is also given in the Output 8.2. In this example, we see there is considerable evidence neither the intercept nor the slope are zero. Inference on the intercept is not particularly useful in this example, but the positive slope on dose and the corresponding small p-value (0.003) provides strong evidence the insecticide is toxic to these insects, and increasing the exposure level is associated with greater levels of mortality.

We can also fit a probit model in **R** by specifying the link = probit in Output 8.3. The logistic link is the default if no link is specified. The slope and intercept each have estimates, standard errors, z statistics, and p-values. We see the slope on dose is positive and achieves an extreme level of statistical significance, leading, again, to the conclusion that higher levels of the insecticide are associated with greater mortality. The parameter estimates for the probit model are very different from those of logistic regression, but, in general, p-values should be comparable. The estimated slopes and intercepts for probit and logistic regressions are not comparable because these are very different models for the binomial p parameter.

What is missing in logistic and probit regression is a sense of the overall model being fitted. The p parameter is not itself a linear function of the exposure. To find p for the fitted logistic regression model, we need to use the relation in (8.4) with the estimated parameters in (8.5). Figure 8.2 plots the models for both the fitted logistic and probit regressions. This graph includes the empirical mortality rates for each of the six jars of beetles, plotted as dots.

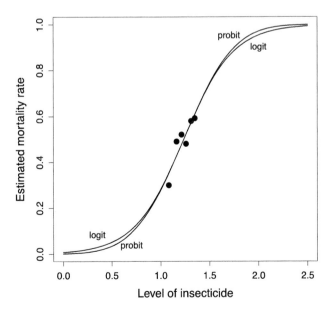

Figure 8.2 Fitted logistic and probit models for the beetle data in Table 8.1. The dots are the empirical mortality rates for each of the six jars.

Output 8.4 Program to draw Fig. 8.2.

```
lb <- glm(resp ~ dose, family = binomial)$coefficients
pb <- glm(resp ~ dose, family = binomial(link = probit))$coefficients
c(lb,pb)                            # print fitted coefficients
dosex <- 0 : 250 / 100              # range of exposure in plot
ln <- exp(lb[1] + lb[2] * dosex)    # numerator of logit
plot(dosex, ln / (1 + ln), type = "l", xlab = "Level of insecticide",
     ylab = "Estimated mortality rate", lwd = 2,
        cex.lab = 1.5)              # plot fitted logit
fitprobit <- pnorm(pb[1] + pb[2] * dosex)   # fitted probit
lines(dosex, fitprobit, type  = "l", lwd = 2)        # add probit to plot
lines(dose, died/N, type = "p", pch = 19, cex = 1.5) # empirical data
text(c(.35, 2, .7, 1.7), c(.08, .9, .035, .95), cex = 1.15,
     labels= c(rep("logit", 2), rep("probit", 2)))
```

Figure 8.2 shows the overall fitted models for the beetle data. Notice the fitted binomial p parameter is always between 0 and 1, for all possible exposure levels of the insecticide. We can also see, at least for the range of exposure levels in these data, there is not much difference between the fitted models for logistic and probit regression models, except in the extreme tails of these models. The probit model is associated with the normal distribution and tends to have shorter tails. That is, the logistic model approaches the limits of 0 and 1 more slowly than those of the probit model for extreme levels of exposure. The **R** code in Output 8.4 was used to produce this figure.

8.4   The New York Mets

Sports news reporting probably involves as many numbers as the business news, and these are eagerly examined by statisticians. Table 8.2 presents the win/loss record on a game-by-game basis of the New York Mets from the beginning of the 2007 baseball season until June 3 of that year.

The accompanying article described a steadily improving record for this team. Was this actually the case? We can use logistic regression to test for an improving or worsening trend. Each game's outcome is a binary-valued outcome: win or loss. Tied games are a rare possibility, and we might have to make up a rule in order to include these. We can use the number of days from the start of the season as the explanatory variable in the same way Dose of insecticide is used in (8.3). A positive or negative estimated slope would be indicative of an increasing or decreasing trend in the team's record.

Is this a valid use of logistic regression? On the surface, the data appears to take the correct form: binary-valued outcomes and an explanatory variable (game number). A closer examination of the way the teams play each other reveals some potential

Table 8.2 Win/loss record of the NY Mets for the 2007 season up to June 3.

Game number:									1	1	1	1	1	1	1	1	1	1	2
1	2	3	4	5	6	7	8	9	0	1	2	3	4	5	6	7	8	9	0
W	W	W	L	L	W	L	W	W	L	W	W	W	L	W	L	W	W	L	L

2	2	2	2	2	2	2	2	2	3	3	3	3	3	3	3	3	3	3	4
1	2	3	4	5	6	7	8	9	0	1	2	3	4	5	6	7	8	9	0
W	W	L	L	W	W	W	W	L	L	W	W	W	L	W	W	L	W	W	W

4	4	4	4	4	4	4	4	4	5	5	5	5	5
1	2	3	4	5	6	7	8	9	0	1	2	3	4
W	L	L	W	L	W	W	W	W	L	W	L	W	L

Source: New York Times.

problems. Remember not all of these games are played against the same opponents. Baseball teams are usually scheduled to host an out-of-town visiting team for a series of several games and then travel to some distant city for a series of several games with another team. The same team is not made up of the same key players from one game to the next because a pitcher needs to rest his arm for a few days after playing. Additional explanatory variables might include whether each of the games played was at home or away and the strength of the opponent at each game. There are statisticians who analyze sports data very carefully and include all of these factors in their models. Exercise 8.2 asks you to perform your own analysis of this data.

8.5 Key Points

Logistic regression is a useful method for studying binomial or binary-valued data. The logit is not a probability, and this concept takes some familiarity before it becomes comfortable. Epidemiologists talk in terms of a change in the odds (or in our case the log-odds) of some outcome. We are not building a linear model of the probability of the outcome, but rather a linear model of the log-odds.

The probit has the same curved shape as the logit. Both produce approximately the same fitted model, although the regression coefficients will be measured on a different scale. Look back at Fig. 8.2 and remind yourself what the model represents. There will not be much difference between the fitted logit and the probit curves unless the probabilities you are measuring are very close to either zero or one.

Use logistic regression to model the p parameter of binomial data. The probit model is another equally good choice. The model in glm looks like the one you used to fit linear models, but here we model the log-odds of the binomial probability through the family or link options. The model notation in glm is similar to the method we used to specify our model in lm for linear models. The binomial response values in glm are two separate columns of values for success and failure. There are a number of useful diagnostic measures explained in Chapter 9.

Are there times when we need to estimate the n parameter of the binomial distribution as well as p? Sometimes we want to estimate the size of a finite population. In Section 1.1, for example, we discussed problems with the census undercount. As another example, suppose we want to estimate the number of homeless people, or the number of persons with HIV in a city. We might need to estimate the fraction p who routinely visit a shelter or clinic but we may also want to estimate the number N who are potential users of these facilities. One way to do this is to first identify individuals and then wait until we see them again, if we ever do. Such surveys are called *mark–recapture* because of their use in wildlife abundance studies. These are specialized statistical methods beyond the scope of the present book but have more recently been used in studies of human populations.

8.6   Exercises

8.1 a. Use the `exp()` function in **R** to estimate the fraction of beetles killed if left unexposed to the insecticide. Can you explain why is this value larger than zero? Look at Fig. 8.2 and notice *negative* doses will also have a nonnegligible proportion of insects killed. Is this a good or bad feature of logistic regression?

   b. Estimate the dose of insecticide to kill 50% of the insects from the results in Output 8.2. Hint: Show logit$(1/2) = 0$. Solve

$$\text{logit}(1/2) = \alpha + \beta \, \text{Dose}$$

   for the Dose using the estimated slope and intercept. This value is referred to as the LD_{50}.

   c. Estimate the dose of insecticide to kill 0.1% of the insects. Would you judge this to be a safe exposure level for humans? Why? For more details on the methods of this exercise, also see Section 8.6.3.

   d. If you were to perform this experiment again, how would you choose doses to answer part (c)? Would you select values of the dose between 1 and 1.5, or would you spread the doses over a wider range?

8.2 Examine the win/loss record given in Table 8.2. Fit a logistic model with the game number as the explanatory x variable. Does it look as though the Mets are losing more games as the season progresses? Is the trend in the earlier games different from the later games?

8.3 The *sex ratio* is the ratio of male to female live births. Usually this is about 51% or slightly more males than females. A lower ratio is sometimes associated with environmental changes such as the presence of endocrine disrupting chemicals.

A report about sex ratios in the Canadian Aamjiwnaang First Nation near Sarnia, Ontario, was published in Mackenzie *et al.* (2005). They identify sex ratios as low as 30% in recent years. Sarnia is near the center of many chemical processing plants and refineries.

a. Obtain the reference

www.ncbi.nlm.nih.gov/pmc/articles/PMC1281269/

and identify the statistical methods used to analyze the data. Are these methods appropriate or not? Do you agree or disagree with the conclusions of the data analysis?

b. How was the data obtained? Comment on the appropriateness of this method.

c. Another report on changes sex ratios in California is given in Smith and Von Behren (2005). The link is

www.ncbi.nlm.nih.gov/pubmed/16286492.

Contrast the data, methods, and conclusions between these separate reports.

8.6.1 A Phase I Clinical Trial in Cancer

One of the dangerous side effects of high-dose chemotherapy is the destruction of beneficial neutrophils, resulting in a condition called neutropenia. A cancer patient may simultaneously be given granulocyte colony-stimulating factor (G-CSF), which encourages neutrophil production and reduces the risk of neutropenia. Abbruzzese *et al.* (1996) report the data in Table 8.3 from cancer patients treated at various doses of topotecan, with and without G-CSF.

Patients may appear more than once in this table because they are typically treated in multiple courses and at different doses. Patients are given sufficient time to recover between courses, so we can usually assume courses are independent of each other. Each course can result in neutropenia or not, so treat the number of courses as the binomial n. The number of neutropenia cases in each group of doses is the binomial distributed number of successes. The binomial p will depend on the dose of topotecan and whether or not G-CSF is used.

Fit a logistic model to explain the incidence of neutropenia in Table 8.3. Is there evidence the risk of neutropenia is nonlinear in the dose of topotecan? Try fitting a logistic regression linear in Dose and Dose^2. Is the use of G-CSF beneficial?

Table 8.3 Topotecan dose, G-CSF use, neutropenia cases, and number of treatment courses in a Phase I clinical trial in cancer.

Dose	G-CSF use?	Neutropenia cases	Treatment courses
2.5	no	0	3
3.0	no	0	3
4.0	no	1	6
5.0	no	1	6
6.25	no	0	3
8.0	no	0	3
10.0	no	1	3
12.5	no	2	6
12.5	yes	1	6
15.0	yes	3	5

One goal of Phase I clinical trials is to estimate a safe dose of the drug being tested. Can you estimate a safe dose for topotecan, with and without G-CSF? The word safe, in this context, usually means a probability of 1 in 6 (or lower) of an adverse experience.

Hint: If $p = 1/6$ then the logit of p is

$$\text{logit}(1/6) = \log \left\{ \frac{1/6}{5/6} \right\} = \log(1/5) = -1.6094$$

and the logistic model specifies

$$\text{logit}(p) = \beta_0 + \beta_1 \text{Dose}.$$

Given the estimates of the slope β_1 and intercept β_0 for this model, we can then solve for the safe dose of topotecan.

8.6.2   Toxoplasmosis in El Salvador

Toxoplasmosis is a disease caused by a parasite. Those with healthy immune systems may experience no ill effects or symptoms. Veterinarians sometimes contract toxoplasmosis from their frequent exposure to cats.

The data in Table 8.4 summarizes the incidence of toxoplasmosis in 11- to 15-year-old children for 34 villages in El Salvador. The table gives the number of children

Table 8.4 Toxoplasmosis cases among children in villages in El Salvador.

Cases	Number tested	Rainfall (mm)	Cases	Number tested	Rainfall (mm)
2	4	1735	3	10	1936
1	5	2000	3	10	1973
2	2	1750	3	5	1800
2	8	1750	7	19	2077
3	6	1920	8	10	1800
7	24	2050	0	1	1830
15	30	1650	4	22	2200
0	1	2000	6	11	1770
0	1	1920	33	54	1770
4	9	2240	5	8	1620
2	12	1756	0	1	1650
8	11	2250	41	77	1796
24	51	1890	7	16	1871
46	82	2063	9	13	2100
23	43	1918	53	75	1834
8	13	1780	3	10	1900
1	6	1976	23	37	2292

Sources: Remington *et al.* (1970) and Efron (1978); data available from https://rdrr.io/cran/rsq/man/toxo.html.

Output 8.5 Code to read the toxoplasmosis data.

```
> tx <- scan(file = "toxoplasmosis.txt")    # read data as a list
> toxo <- data.frame(NULL)                   # initialize data frame
> while (length(tx) > 0)
+ {
+    toxo <- rbind(toxo, tx[1:3])             # append new row to the end
+    tx <- tx[-(1:3)]                         # remove these values
+ }
> colnames(toxo) <- c("pos", "tested", "rain")
> toxo                                        # always look at it
    pos tested rain
1    2      4 1735
2    3     10 1936
3    1      5 2000
      . . .
33   1      6 1976
34  23     37 2292
> resp <- cbind(toxo$pos,
+                  toxo$tested - toxo$pos)    # response for logistic reg'n.
> resp
       [,1] [,2]
  [1,]   2    2
  [2,]   3    7
  [3,]   1    4
      . . .

 [33,]   1    5
 [34,]  23   14
```

---

tested (the binomial **n** parameter), the number of these who were found positive for toxoplasmosis (the binomial response *y*) and the annual rainfall (in millimeters) for each village.

The data is arranged with more than one observation per line so you can use the code in Output 8.5 to read it and create the response vector for glm. Fit a linear logistic model using annual rainfall to explain the rate of toxoplasmosis. Does the incidence increase or decrease with rainfall? Is there evidence more children were tested in villages with greater rainfall? What does this say about how the data was collected?

Fit a logistic model with polynomial terms in rainfall up to the third power. That is, for each village,

$$\text{logit}(p) = \beta_0 + \beta_1 \text{rain} + \beta_2 \text{rain}^2 + \beta_3 \text{rain}^3 .$$

You should first rescale the rainfall observations by dividing these by 1000. (What happens if you don't?) Does this cubic model explain the data any better than the model with only a linear term? What does this tell you about the effect of rainfall on the risk of toxoplasmosis? Does a graph of this fitted cubic function generally increase in rainfall? How does it differ from a straight line?

8.6.3   Estimation of the ED_{01}

Government agencies are charged with identifying safe exposure levels of toxic chemicals in our air and water. Workers who routinely come in to contact with these chemicals also have to be protected against toxic levels. Healthcare workers usually wear photographic-sensitive badges to measure their cumulative exposure to X-ray radiation. How are these safe exposure levels established? The regulatory process is rather lengthy, but we can sometimes provide a rough estimate using simple methods.

The data given in Table 8.5 was generated, in part, to see how well the logit and probit models can be used to estimate extremely low probabilities of developing liver cancer when exposed to a known carcinogen. Very large numbers of female mice were exposed to low levels of the chemical in order to estimate the dose–response at such low levels.

The *effective dose* of a compound resulting in 50% of the outcome is abbreviated as ED_{50}. Similarly, the ED_{01} is the exposure level with a 1% effective rate. Sometimes these may be written as the LD_{01} for an estimated 1% *lethal dose*, or even the LD_{001} for a 0.1% lethal dose.

Table 8.5 The upper number is the number of mice developing liver cancer, and the lower number is the number exposed to the combination of dose and duration.

Months on study	Dose in parts 10^{-4}							
	0.0	0.30	0.35	0.45	0.60	0.75	1.00	1.50
9	0	1	1	0	0	0	1	1
	199	147	76	52	345	186	168	169
12	0	1	2	1	2	0	3	2
	164	151	27	14	283	153	149	152
14	1	1	0	2	1	0	1	1
	133	42	25	14	243	124	127	127
15	0	1	1	0	3	1	5	1
	115	75	35	20	203	109	99	100
16	1	2	2	3	6	7	2	7
	205	66	61	304	287	193	100	110
17	0	4	5	6	8	9	3	1
	153	69	443	302	230	166	85	82
18	6	34	20	15	13	17	19	24
	555	2014	1102	550	411	382	213	211
24	20	164	128	98	118	118	76	126
	762	2109	1361	888	758	587	297	314
33+	17	135	72	42	30	37	22	9
	100	445	100	103	67	75	31	11

Source: Farmer *et al.* (1979).

This table summarizes the outcome of a very large number of female mice continuously exposed to the carcinogen 2-acetylaminofluorene (2-AAF) at very low doses for specific periods of time. The mice were then sacrificed and examined by pathologists for the presence of tumors in their livers.

Use this data to see how well the logit and probit models estimate the cancer rates in mice at extremely low levels of exposure. Notice the unexposed mice were not entirely disease-free. Does the logit of the cancer rate appear to be linear in dose? Are the effects of dose and duration additive, or does there appear to be an interaction between these two risk factors?

Try to estimate the ED_{01} using your fitted model. Does your model produce a reasonable estimate? Next try deleting some of the data at the lowest doses and see how accurately your model fits the missing values.

What would happen if you consider doing a similar analysis, estimating the ED_{01} using the beetle data given in Table 8.1? It would be relatively easy for us to take the fitted logit or probit model and use the method in Section 8.6.1 to estimate the ED_{01}. This would provide a quick and inexpensive estimate.

What is wrong with following this procedure for the beetle data? A quick look at Fig. 8.2 reveals there is very little data anywhere near the ED_{01}. Most of the data is centered near the middle or ED_{50} of this figure. It is worth repeating the following advice.

Extrapolate at your peril.

Estimating properties about an event occurring only 1% of the time will require a large and expensive experiment and will not provide the outcome 99% of the time. There is no shortcut for quality data in order to yield a reasonable estimate. Table 8.5 gives data on over 20,000 mice. Obtaining this data took a great amount of time and planning.

8.6.4 Super Bowl XXXVIII

This football game was played in Houston on Sunday, February 1, 2004, between the New England Patriots and the Carolina Panthers. The Patriots won 32 to 29 on a play in the last four seconds of the game.

Notice both teams were in possession of the ball the same number of times (13). Did one team begin significantly closer to its goal, on average? You might use a t-test to answer this question. Intuitively, the closer the team begins to its goal, the more likely it is to score. Is this the case with the present data? Here are some other questions you might use logistic regression to answer. Raise any other points you want to about this data.

- Do shorter distances to the goal increase the probability of a team scoring?
- Is there a trend for more scoring later in the game? The time of each play is not given here, but we can use the drive number as an indication of how early or late

Table 8.6 Summary of each drive in Super Bowl XXXVIII. Columns are: team with the ball (N: New England Patriots; C: Carolina Panthers); drive or possession number; starting distance in yards to their goal line; indication of a scoring drive (0 = no, 1 = yes).

Team	Drive	Dist	Score?	Team	Drive	Dist	Score?
N	1	48	0	N	2	62	0
N	3	49	0	N	4	68	0
N	5	76	0	N	6	20	1
N	7	77	1	N	8	75	0
N	9	90	0	N	10	71	1
N	11	73	0	N	12	68	1
N	13	60	1 ←—The game-winning drive				
C	1	78	0	C	2	79	0
C	3	89	0	C	4	92	0
C	5	62	0	C	6	72	0
C	7	95	1	C	8	52	1
C	9	59	0	C	10	90	0
C	11	81	1	C	12	90	1
C	13	80	1				

Reported by the *New York Times*, February 2, 2004.

each event occurred. Why do you think there might be more scoring later in the game?

• Is there an interaction indicating one team was increasingly likely to score later in the game? What does this show?
• Is the effect of the distance to the goal smaller or greater than the later-in-the-game effect? What does this tell us?

Running a television ad during the Superbowl is very expensive. The price was approximately $2 million for a 30-second message during this game. If you were an advertiser, where would you want your ad to appear: early in the game when your audience is still alert; at half-time; or toward the end, when the earlier audience members may have either changed channels or become more engaged by a close ending? There was a joke that all sewers across the United States would overflow at half-time as millions of Americans simultaneously went to the bathroom. Comment on the element of uncertainty associated with these three different time points in the game.

When all the binomial *n* parameters are equal to one, as in this example, we can denote the responses as a single column of success/failures as in this example:

```
sb <- read.table(file = "Superbowl.txt", header = T)
glm(score ~ drive + start + team, data = sb, family = binomial)
```

and **R** will build an indicator variable for you to identify the team.

9 Diagnostics for Logistic Regression

Let's review what was covered in Chapter 8. The logistic model is a useful method to examine the p parameter of binomial data. In order to keep our estimate of p between 0 and 1, we need to model functions of p. The log-odds or $\log(p/(1-p))$ is called the *logit* and is modeled as a linear function of covariates. There are other variations on this idea. The *probit* models the cumulative normal distribution as a linear function of covariates. Both the logit and probit were designed to keep estimates of p between 0 and 1. The `link=probit` option in `glm` can be used to fit the probit model. There is little difference between the two fitted models, as we see when we look at Fig. 8.2.

Output 8.2 provides statistical significance of the regression slope, but it does not tell us much about how well the model fits or even whether it is appropriate. In this chapter we want to discuss several diagnostic measures available to detect outliers and observations with high influence. Many of these have a parallel measure in linear regression, discussed in Chapter 5. Before we get to that, let's introduce another example.

9.1 A Larger Example

The data in Table 9.1 is a list of men with prostate cancer. If the cancer is localized, then the disease is still in an early stage. A localized cancer also means the treatment is more likely to be successful. Prostate cancer is more serious if it has already spread to the lymph nodes. Surgery is needed to determine if the spread has already happened. It would be better if we could find a less intrusive estimator of the risk of nodal involvement. Such a model would spare an unnecessary surgery for those men at lowest risk and also alert the physician to those patients at high risk.

The outcome (y) variable is nodal involvement and is binary valued. Binary-valued covariates (X-ray, stage, and grade) have been coded so the "0" values are the less serious status. Age and serum acid phosphatase are continuous measures.

Questions to ask from this data: What are useful predictors of nodal status? Are the explanatory variables independent of each other, or are these correlated with each other? What does this say about their individual and collective use as diagnostic measures? Are there any outliers or highly influential observations with undue effect on the fitted model?

Table 9.1 Nodal involvement in prostate cancer patients. The six columns are: X-ray status; stage of the cancer; grade of the tumor; age of the patient; serum acid phosphatase; and nodal involvement (1 = yes, 0 = no).

X-ray	Stage	Grade	Age	Acid	Nodes	X-ray	Stage	Grade	Age	Acid	Nodes
0	0	0	66	48	0	0	0	0	68	56	0
0	0	0	66	50	0	0	0	0	56	52	0
0	0	0	58	50	0	0	0	0	60	49	0
1	0	0	65	46	0	1	0	0	60	62	0
0	0	1	50	56	1	1	0	0	49	55	0
0	0	0	61	62	0	0	0	0	58	71	0
0	0	0	51	65	0	1	0	1	67	67	1
0	0	1	67	47	0	0	0	0	51	49	0
0	0	1	56	50	0	0	0	0	60	78	0
0	0	0	52	83	0	0	0	0	56	98	0
0	0	0	67	52	0	0	0	0	63	75	0
0	0	1	59	99	1	0	0	0	64	187	0
1	0	0	61	136	1	0	0	0	56	82	1
0	1	1	64	40	0	0	1	0	61	50	0
0	1	1	64	50	0	0	1	0	63	40	0
0	1	1	52	55	0	0	1	1	66	59	0
1	1	0	58	48	1	1	1	1	57	51	1
0	1	0	65	49	1	0	1	1	65	48	0
1	1	1	59	63	0	0	1	0	61	102	0
0	1	0	53	76	0	0	1	0	67	95	0
0	1	1	53	66	0	1	1	1	65	84	1
1	1	1	50	81	1	1	1	1	60	76	1
0	1	1	45	70	1	1	1	1	56	78	1
0	1	0	46	70	1	0	1	0	67	67	1
0	1	0	63	82	1	0	1	1	57	67	1
1	1	0	51	72	1	1	1	0	64	89	1
1	1	1	68	126	1						

Available as nodal in the boot library.

There is a large overlap between logistic regression modeling and multivariate linear regression discussed in Chapter 5. Many of the diagnostic measures have the same names and roles. Even the **R** code should look familiar in Output 9.1.

The summary and influence statements will produce familiar diagnostics we saw with linear regression but some of these need to be interpreted differently for logistic regression. Selected material from summary includes Output 9.2, a familiar table of fitted parameter values, their standard errors, and tests of statistical significance. In this case, xray, stage, and acid values appear to offer a good amount of explanatory value.

The model specification for glm in Output 9.1 is different from most of the examples given in the previous chapter. Every man listed in Table 9.1 is different from all others, with his own unique set of risk factors. For the binomial data in this example, every N parameter is equal to one. When this is the case, the response values in glm

---

Output 9.1 **R** syntax to obtain diagnostics in logistic regression in nodal cancer.

```
> # Nodal involvement in prostate cancer
> pc <- read.table(file = "nodal.txt", header = T)
> pc[1:3,]                        # remember to look at a few
  xray stage grade age acid node
1   0     0     0  66   48    0
2   0     0     0  68   56    0
3   0     0     0  66   50    0
> pc.logit <- glm(node ~ xray + stage + grade + age + acid,
+                 data = pc, family = binomial)
> pc.sum <- summary(pc.logit)
> pc.inf <- influence(pc.logit)
> labels(pc.inf)                  # names of influence diagnostics
[1] "hat"          "coefficients" "sigma"        "dev.res"
[5] "pear.res"
> pc.inf$hat[1:3]                 # look at a few hat values
         1          2          3
0.03016299 0.03273938 0.03061336
> pc.inf$dev.res[1:3]             # a few deviance residuals
         1          2          3
-0.2638030 -0.2711911 -0.2701881
```

Output 9.2 Part of the summary for the prostate cancer example.

```
Coefficients:
            Estimate Std. Error z value Pr(>|z|)
(Intercept)  0.06180    3.45992   0.018   0.9857
xray         2.04534    0.80718   2.534   0.0113 *
stage        1.56410    0.77401   2.021   0.0433 *
grade        0.76142    0.77077   0.988   0.3232
age         -0.06926    0.05788  -1.197   0.2314
acid         0.02434    0.01316   1.850   0.0643 .
---
Signif. codes:  0 '***' 0.001 '**' 0.01 '*' 0.05 '.' 0.1 ' ' 1
```

---

are specified as a single column of values, signifying the success or failure of each individual. A similar remark was made in Exercise 8.6.4 and Section 8.4.

9.2   Residuals for Logistic Regression

We have already seen the importance of examining residuals in identifying exceptional observations in the data. Despite their critical role in linear regression models, there are different definitions of residuals in logistic regression. There is a simple explanation for this. In linear regression with normally distributed errors, one of the fundamental assumptions is the model errors have a constant variance. See Section 4.4 for a review of this. Similarly, we fit linear regression models using least squares of these residual values. So, in linear regression, we rely on residuals to both fit the model and then tell us how well it explains the data. In logistic regression there are several definitions of residuals, each interesting in its own way.

So, for example, we could just use the definition of residuals from linear regression, namely, the difference between observed and expected. These *raw residuals* are defined as

$$\text{Raw residual} = \text{Observed} - \text{Expected} = y - n\hat{p},$$

where $\hat{p}$ is the value fitted by logistic regression.

In **R** for the prostate cancer example, we can construct these using

```
phat <- pc.logit$fitted.values      # fitted p parameters
raw.resid <- pc$node - phat          # observed - expected
```

where pc.logit is the output from glm.

What is wrong with looking at the raw residuals? A problem with logistic regression for binary-valued data is the binomial distribution does not have a constant variance, unlike the assumption we make for linear regression with normally distributed errors. The formula for the binomial variance is $np(1 - p)$, given in (2.3). Specifically, when the p parameter is close to either 0 or 1 then all of the observations are likely to be failures or successes, respectively, with little variability. So the variance is a function of the fitted value.

A simple correction to the raw residual is to divide each of these by their estimated standard error. These are the *Pearson residuals* or the *chi-squared residuals*. These are defined as

$$\text{Pearson residual} = \frac{y - n\hat{p}}{\sqrt{n\hat{p}(1 - \hat{p})}},$$

and obtained as pear.res from the influence program in **R**.

An example for the prostate cancer data appears in Output 9.1. Recall, for prostate cancer example, all n parameters are equal to one.

The Pearson residuals are plotted against the observation number in Fig. 9.1. Plots against the observation number are often called *index plots*.

This also leads us to raise the question: How does **R** fit the regression parameters in logistic regression? Unlike the residual sums of squares minimized in Section 3.2 on linear regression, estimates of the regression coefficients are obtained by minimizing the *deviance* function, which is defined as

$$\text{Deviance} = 2\sum_i \left[y_i \log\left\{\frac{y_i}{n_i p_i}\right\} + (n_i - y_i)\log\left\{\frac{n_i - y_i}{n_i(1 - p_i)}\right\}\right]. \tag{9.1}$$

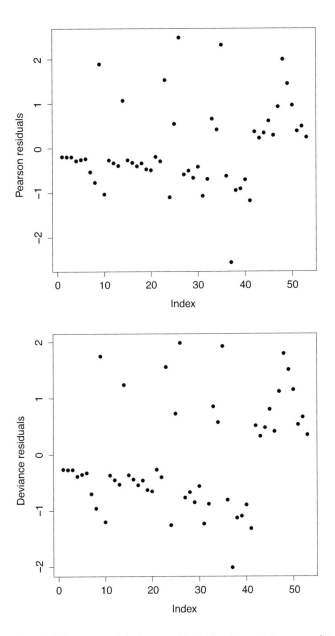

Figure 9.1 Pearson and deviance residuals for the prostate cancer data.

Where are the regression parameters in this expression? It is not clear at first glance, but recall the p parameters are functions of the regression coefficients when we write

$$\text{logit}(p) = \log(p/(1-p)) = \alpha + \beta_1 x_1 + \cdots$$

and then use this in the deviance (9.1).

The values of α, β_1, ... minimizing the deviance are also called the *maximum like-lihood estimates*. The deviance function behaves much like the Pearson chi-squared statistic, and these statistics play similar roles.

Just as the Pearson residuals can be squared and added together to give us the Pearson chi-squared statistic, there are also *deviance residuals* whose sum of squared values give the deviance statistic. These are defined as

$$\text{Deviance residual} = \pm\sqrt{2}\left[y_i \log\left\{\frac{y_i}{n_i \hat{p}_i}\right\} + (n_i - y_i)\log\left\{\frac{n_i - y_i}{n_i(1 - \hat{p}_i)}\right\}\right]^{1/2},$$

where the $\pm$ sign is determined by whether the observed y_i is greater or less than the expected $n_i \hat{p}_i$.

These residuals have the property

$$\text{Deviance} = \sum_i (\text{Deviance residual})^2.$$

Deviance residuals are obtained in **R** as dev.res from the influence function in Output 9.1.

The Pearson and deviance residuals are plotted against the observation number in Fig. 9.1 and there is almost no difference in the appearance of these two figures. Very few of either of these types of residuals are greater than ± 2 in magnitude, indicating there are few outliers.

There are some things about these two residual plots not quite right, however. Notice how the residuals form two clouds of values above and below the zero value line but do not actually touch it. This is even more striking in the plot of deviance residuals. Why does the residual plot take this peculiar shape?

Even though the residuals for this model have a mean of 0 and a standard deviation close to 1, there is no reason for these to behave as though they were sampled from a normal, bell-shaped distribution. Specifically, in this example, recall all of the binomial n parameters are equal to 1. The binomial response variables y will only take on the values 0 or 1, and the estimated $\hat{p}$ parameter can take on any value between 0 and 1.

The raw residuals are defined as $y - n\hat{p}$ and all of the $n = 1$ in this case. When $y = 1$ the estimated $\hat{p}$ will always underestimate the response. Similarly, when $y = 0$, the estimate $\hat{p}$ will always overestimate the response. In other words, the cloud of residuals above the zero line correspond to values of $y = 1$, and the residuals below the zero line are associated with $y = 0$ responses. The standardization of the raw residuals by their estimated standard error will change the scale of the residuals and actually push them further away from 0. See Exercise 9.2 for an explanation of this.

You may have also noticed a decreasing trend in the residual plots of Fig. 9.1 for these data. Why is this the case? Hints are given Exercise 9.3.

Does this mean residuals are not useful in logistic regression? No. Residuals are still useful, especially in identifying poorly fitting outliers in the data. The difficulty

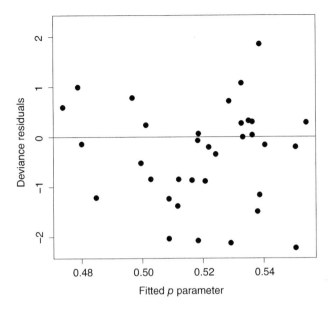

Figure 9.2 Deviance residuals and fitted $\hat{p}$ for the toxoplasmosis data of Section 8.6.2.

arises when all of the binomial N parameters are equal to 1 or other small counts. Then we cannot expect the responses to behave approximately as normally distributed. The residuals may not take values close to 0 even in a well-fitting model.

As another example of residuals, look back at the toxoplasmosis example of Section 8.6.2. In this example, a small number of villages had only $n = 1$ or 2 children tested, but most villages had much larger values. Let us fit a model in which the logit of the risk of infection in each village is expressible as a linear function of rainfall.

The deviance residuals are plotted against the fitted $\hat{p}$ values in Fig. 9.2. In this figure we see the residuals appear to be reasonably distributed close to the zero line and there are few large outliers to point out. The residuals on this figure behave more as we would expect because most of the binomial n parameters are greater than 1.

A careful look at the residual plots does exhibit a slight "U"-shape. The positive residuals only appear at the extreme values of the estimated p parameter. Does this provide evidence of a nonlinear effect of rainfall? Section 8.6.2 suggests a model to address this.

9.3 Influence in Logistic Regression

Many of the diagnostic measures for logistic regression have a direct parallel and are borrowed from linear regression. For example, there is a hat diagonal for logistic regression similar to the influence measure we saw in Section 5.3. This measure is called hat in Output 9.1. The index plot of the hat diagonal appears in Fig. 9.3.

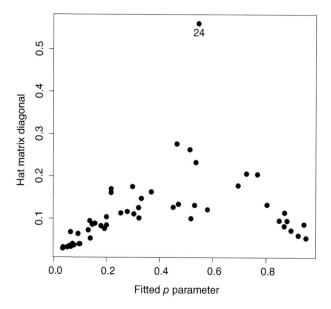

Figure 9.3 Hat matrix diagonal for the prostate cancer data.

Figure 9.3 shows most of the patients have reasonable influence in the logistic regression, but observation 24 stands out from the rest. Recall the hat diagonal only indicates outliers among the explanatory values, not the response. In Fig. 9.1 we see this observation has a negative residual but this is not extreme. This observation appears to follow the form of the model, but something is not quite right. The hat matrix diagonal points this observation out to us, but it does not explain it.

To find out, we need to introduce the other diagnostics. Useful diagnostics can be produced with the **R** program

$$\texttt{blr\_plot\_diag\_influence(pc.logit)}$$

in the `blorr` library.

The `pc.logit` is the output of the `glm` program, produced in Output 9.1. Figure 9.4 is produced by this program. Additional useful figures are produced by

$$\texttt{blr\_plot\_diag\_fit(pc.logit)}$$

which plots diagnostics by fitted value and

$$\texttt{blr\_plot\_diag\_leverage(pc.logit)}$$

which plots diagnostic values by their hat value.

Two popular diagnostic measures are c and $\bar{c}$. Together, these two measures are also referred to as the *confidence interval displacement*. These combine the Pearson residual and the hat diagonal. They are calculated as

$$c = (\text{Pearson residual})^2 \times \text{hat}/(1 - \text{hat})^2$$

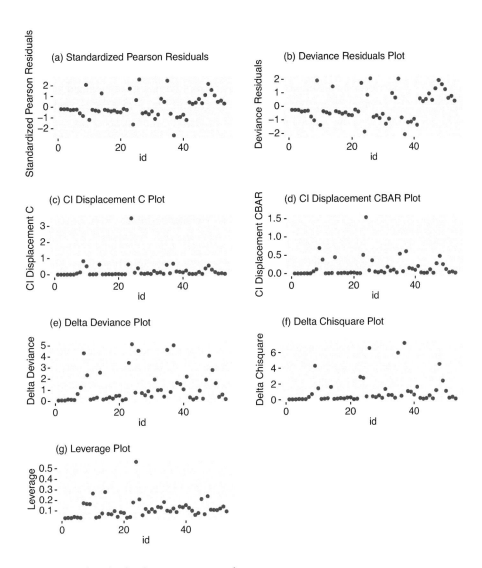

Figure 9.4 Index plot for the prostate cancer data.

and

$$\bar{c} = (\text{Pearson residual})^2 \times \text{hat}/(1 - \text{hat}),$$

respectively.

Index plots of c and $\bar{c}$ for the prostate cancer data are given in Figs. 9.4 (c) and (d). These look much like a plot of the hat diagonal in Fig. 9.3. As is the case of the hat diagnostic, plots of c and $\bar{c}$ indicate observation 24 is unusual but do not help explain why this is the case.

The remaining diagnostics for logistic regression derive from jackknife methods. Recall from Section 5.4 the jackknife is a general technique which omits an observation and then refits the model without the observation. The new fitted model is then compared to the original model fitted from all of the data.

Specifically, the `difchisq` and `difdev` are the change in Pearson chi-squared and the deviance functions when individual observations are deleted and then the model is refitted. These two measures are typically used to identify outliers because they indicate how much the overall fit is altered when observations are omitted. These statistics are calculated as

$$\texttt{difchisq} = \bar{c} / \text{hat} = (\text{Pearson residual})^2 / (1 - \text{hat})$$

and

$$\texttt{difdev} = (\text{Deviance residual})^2 + \bar{c},$$

respectively, for each observation.

The index plot of `difdev` and `difchisq` appear in Figs. 9.4 (e) and (f). These two plots are almost identical. Observation 24 is not remarkable in these graphs. Several other observations have larger values of `difdev`. None of these appear to stand out either. To determine the problem with observation 24, we have to introduce other diagnostics.

The `dfbeta` diagnostics are introduced in Section 5.4 and show how much the estimated regression coefficients change when individual observations are deleted and the model is refitted. The same idea applied to linear regression also works for logistic regression. There will be a `dfbeta` measure for every term in the logistic regression model, including the intercept.

The `dfbeta` is specific to each regression coefficient. An unusual `dfbeta` for one estimated regression coefficient may not be remarkable for another. Most plots of the `dfbetas` for the prostate cancer example in Fig. 9.5 are not remarkable, but one really stands out. The index plot for the serum acid phosphatase `dfbeta` is given in Fig. 9.5 (e).

In this diagnostic plot we can easily see how observation 24 is different from the others. Now we know something is unusual about the serum acid level for this subject. If we look back at the original data in Table 9.1, we see his serum acid level is 187, a value much higher than for any other individual. This extremely high acid level is the source of the influence for this cancer patient, revealing the problem.

In this section, we described a number of diagnostic measures for logistic regression. Not all of these will be useful all of the time, of course. Residuals are important and identify poorly fitting observations but are not helpful when the binomial n parameters are equal to one.

Some diagnostics such as the hat and `dfbeta` are used to identify unusual values among the explanatory variables. In the example of the prostate cancer patients, we saw other measures, such as c and $\bar{c}$, are useful for identifying unusual observations. Other measures, such as `difdev` and `difchisq`, may miss these influential observations if the model fits them well. Finally, the `dfbetas` are specific to each term in the model. Taken together, these diagnostics are helpful in identifying influential and unusual observations in our data.

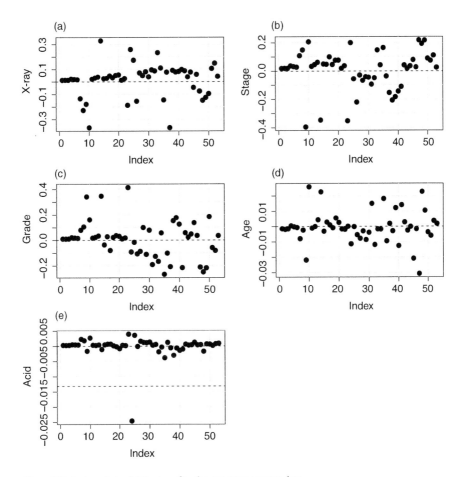

Figure 9.5 Index plot of dfbetas for the prostate cancer data.

9.4 Exercises

9.1 Suppose we are modeling the binomial probability of failure $1 - p$ rather than the probability p of success. If we accidentally ran the program modeling success, do we need to run the program again? What can be done to fix the problem?

Hint: The log of a reciprocal is the negative of the log. That is, $\log(1/x) = -\log(x)$. Describe the relationship between

$$\log\left\{\frac{p}{1-p}\right\}$$

and

$$\log\left\{\frac{1-p}{p}\right\}.$$

What should we do to the estimated regression coefficients in the logistic model?

9.2 When the N parameters are all equal to one in a logistic regression, are the raw residuals closer to 0 or further away from zero than the Pearson residuals? Hint: What can you say about the denominator of the Pearson residuals?

9.3 Notice the trend in the residual plots in Fig. 9.1, especially among the negative residuals. Can you explain this? What does the horizontal axis in this plot represent? Could this be a risk factor for nodal involvement? Why do you think this might be the case? Run a logistic regression model and see if case number is a useful and statistically significant measure of risk of nodal involvement.

9.4.1   Statistics in the News: Sex and Violins

In a news article about a reverse sex-discrimination case, a male violinist was suing a major symphony orchestra claiming, among other things, there were too many female violinists. The *New York Times* printed the data in Table 9.2 detailing the gender breakdown of the string sections of several major US symphony orchestras. The data was obtained from the individual orchestras' web pages.

An opening for a position in a major symphony orchestra may bring hundreds of applicants from many countries. To ensure fairness to these performers, most modern symphony auditions are conducted anonymously. Orchestras will usually audition players for their positions behind screens so they can be heard but not seen. The players' identities are usually not known by those doing the hiring until after a decision has been reached. The orchestras will often go so far as to provide thick carpeting so even the performer's footsteps cannot be heard behind the screen.

Possible statistical analysis includes the following.

a. Show female players appear more often in the higher-pitched instruments. The order of deeper pitch is violin, viola, 'cello, bass. Notice, for example, there are almost no female bass players. Do you think smaller or larger hands may be advantageous for some instruments?

Table 9.2 Members of major US symphony orchestra string sections, listed by sex.

Name	Total	Violin M	Violin F	Viola M	Viola F	'Cello M	'Cello F	Bass M	Bass F
Chicago Symphony	68	14	20	10	4	10	1	9	0
LA Philharmonic	66	15	17	8	5	11	1	9	0
Cleveland Orchestra	65	16	17	7	5	9	2	9	0
New York Philharmonic	65	13	20	5	7	5	6	7	2
Philadelphia Orchestra	65	21	11	8	4	9	3	9	0
Cincinnati Symphony	63	16	17	8	4	7	3	8	0
Boston Symphony	62	13	18	7	5	9	1	9	0
National Symphony	62	14	17	4	7	9	3	8	0
Baltimore Symphony	58	18	10	6	6	5	5	8	0

Data reported by the *New York Times* from the orchestras' web pages.

Output 9.3 Program to read and reformat the orchestra data.

```
> or <- read.table(file = "symphony.txt")
> no <- dim(or)[1]                          # number of orchestras
> F <- c(or[ ,4], or[, 6], or[, 8], or[, 10])   # Female counts
> M <- c(or[, 3], or[, 5], or[, 7], or[, 9])    # Male counts
> inst <- rep(c("violin", "viola", "cello", "bass"), each = no)
> name <- rep(or[, 1], 4)                    # orchestra numbers
> size <- or[,2]                             # size of each
> orch <- data.frame(cbind(F, M, size, inst, name))
> orch
    F  M size    inst name
1  20 14   68 violin    3
2  17 15   66 violin    6
3  17 16   65 violin    5
        .  .  .  .
```

---

b. Does the percentage of female membership change with size of the string section? Is the total number (size) of string players a useful covariate?

c. Which orchestras more prone to males or females predominating?

The outline of a suggested program to reformat the data is given in Output 9.3. Run this program and see how the data is reformatted. Use this program as the basis of your examination of these data using logistic regression. As always, be on the lookout for outliers and points of high influence.

9.4.2   Glove Use among Nurses

In an effort to increase the use of gloves among pediatric nurses, Friedland *et al.* (1992) conducted a study conducted in the emergency department of an inner-city pediatric hospital. Without their knowledge, the nurses were observed during a vascular procedure and the observers recorded how often they used gloves. Observations were made at four time points: before a training period and at 1, 2, and 5 months following the training period. For each of the four periods, Table 9.3 gives the number of times each nurse was observed to perform the procedure (N) and how many of these times he or she wore gloves (y). The number of years of experience for each nurse is also given.

Notice the longitudinal nature of the data. The observations were collected over a period of time. It might help to review the discussion of methods for longitudinal data given in Section 6.5 and Exercise 6.6 for the approach in a specific example. In this present example, the outcomes (gloved or ungloved procedures) are binary valued, but most of the same principles remain.

Even though each nurse was observed at up to four different time periods, let us treat these as independent binomial experiments. Create a binary-valued indicator variable equal to 0 at the first period and 1 for all posttraining periods. Use this indicator in a logistic regression to see if there was a (marginal) difference in the use

Table 9.3 Glove use among nurses for four observation periods. Missing values are indicated by blank spaces.

Years of experience	Period 1		Period 2		Period 3		Period 4	
	obs	gloved	obs	gloved	obs	gloved	obs	gloved
15	2	1	7	6	1	1		
2	2	1	6	5	11	10	9	9
3	5	5	13	13	8	7	15	14
10	2	0	2	2	2	2	5	4
20	12	0	2	2	3	3	3	0
8	3	0	8	8	3	2	4	2
9	4	4	4	4				
4	4	0	4	4	2	1		
15	2	0	3	2	1	1	2	1
8	6	1	1	1	2	2		
8	3	0	4	3	8	6	2	
2	2	0	3	3	8	8	5	5
5	1	0						
15	1	0	3	3				
3	1	1	2	2	1	1	1	1
14	1	0					1	1
14			2	2	3	3	1	1
8			1	1	1	1	1	1
3			2	1				
6			1	1				
3			1	1				
1					2	2		
6							1	0

Source: DASL, https://dasl.datadescription.com/.

of gloves before and after the training period. Does the (marginal) rate of glove use increase or decrease with years of experience? Can you interpret this in simple terms? Look at the interaction between this pre/post indicator and period to see if there was a trend in the posttraining period. Is there evidence whether this posttraining trend is the same regardless of the experience of the nurse? Again, interpret this finding. Use the logistic regression diagnostics to identify outliers or influential observations.

Create an indicator variable for more or fewer than five years' experience. Is there a relationship between the number of observed procedures and this simple measure of experience? Interpret this finding. Does this mean the procedure was performed more often by some nurses, or perhaps some nurses were more likely to be observed and their data recorded?

In a transitional approach to this data, see if there is evidence that individual behavior was changed by the training. Specifically, did individuals with a low frequency of glove use before training change their behavior after training? To answer this question, we might classify every nurse's pretraining glove use as above or below 50%, and then classify their posttraining as above or below 50%. Tabulate the frequencies of these individuals in a 2×2 table. Look at the separate 2×2 tables for those whose experience is above and below five years. Is there a difference in these two frequency tables?

There are a large number of missing values in Table 9.3. These are indicated by blank spaces where data values should be. Missing values are common and play an important part in longitudinal data. Was the frequency of missing observations related to years of experience? Were the missing values more likely in pretraining or post training for more or less experienced nurses? Can you explain this? In Section 6.5 we describe a method called *last value carried forward* to fill in missing values. Does this technique change the conclusions for any of the other questions in this exercise?

9.4.3   Statistics in Sports: Pittsburgh Steelers' Rushing Game

In Table 9.4 we are given a history of the Pittsburgh Steelers for 21 years, under the direction of three different coaches. This includes a win/loss record for each year. *Rushing attempts* indicates the number of running plays. These are not listed as absolute numbers but instead given as ranks among all teams for each year. Similarly,

Table 9.4 Pittsburgh Steelers' rushing records.

| | Games | | Rank of | | |
| | | | Rushing | Rushing | |
Year	Won	Lost	attempts	yards	Coach
1988	5	11	13	6	Chuck Noll
1989	9	7	11	18	Chuck Noll
1990	9	7	14	13	Chuck Noll
1991	7	9	16	17	Chuck Noll
1992	11	5	2	4	Bill Cowher
1993	9	7	5	6	Bill Cowher
1994	12	4	2	1	Bill Cowher
1995	11	5	5	2	Bill Cowher
1996	10	6	2	2	Bill Cowher
1997	11	5	1	1	Bill Cowher
1998	7	9	8	7	Bill Cowher
1999	6	10	5	10	Bill Cowher
2000	9	7	2	4	Bill Cowher
2001	13	3	1	1	Bill Cowher
2002	10	5	3	9	Bill Cowher
2003	6	10	16	31	Bill Cowher
2004	15	1	1	2	Bill Cowher
2005	11	5	1	5	Bill Cowher
2006	8	8	14	10	Bill Cowher
2007	10	6	3	3	Mike Tomlin
2008	12	4	9	23	Mike Tomlin

Reported by the *New York Times*, January 11, 2009.

the number of yards attained is given as the rank compared with all other teams. Of course, each year's data represents the same team in name only, because most players' careers are relatively short. The coaches are working with different players from year to year. The number of teams has changed, as well.

Some would argue rushing, as opposed to passing, is a more conservative strategy. Passing, or throwing the ball, has a higher risk of failure, but more yards are gained when it succeeds. In some years there are changes in the rules favoring either passing or rushing, so the overall strategy of the game has changed over time. Similarly, the number of rushing plays is not as useful as the rank of plays attempted when compared with other teams. Let us use logistic regression to see how the rushing game affects the overall win/loss record for this team.

Is there an association of rushing and yards achieved with the win/loss record? Is there a difference between the three coaches? Do these coaches have a different emphasis on rushing? Are they more successful at it? Has the reliance of rushing plays changed over the years? Is there an interaction between yards attempted and plays run? Are the running plays more successful in some years?

Look for influence and outliers. What was so unusual about the 2003 season? Notice the years under coach Mike Tomlin are influential. The earliest years are influential as well. Why is that?

9.4.4   Climate Records in Washington, DC

Part of the argument about climate change involves the gradual nature of the change. We sense an obvious change in the seasons but the effects of climate change are only visible over many years of careful observation. Good data is needed and should be subjected to careful statistical analysis to identify any trends.

We collected the data in Table 9.5 from the National Weather Service. In many cities, the historical weather data was originally collected in the downtown area but later moved to an airport in the suburbs. In such cities, this might create a downward bias in recorded temperatures over time. For this example, we chose the data continuously monitored at the National Weather Service Forecast office in Baltimore/Washington.

For every calendar day of the year, this table includes normal ranges, rainfall, and extremes, as well as the years in which the extremes occurred. In this exercise we concentrate on extremes in temperature for Washington.

Specifically, we ask whether the record highs occurred before or after the record lows. If there is no trend or change over the years covered by these data then these record values are equally likely to occur in either order, i.e. the record highs are equally likely to appear before or after record lows.

A simple summary of these data was described in Exercise 2.11. In that exercise, we noted in these data, out of 365 calendar days (excluding the leap year) there were 291 days in which the warmest recorded temperature occurred after the coldest recorded value. This is strong statistical evidence against a binomial model with parameter

Table 9.5 Temperature and climate records for Washington, DC, for each calendar day.

A		B		C		D		E		F		G		H	
1	01	44	29	0.09	0.1	69	2005	17	1918	-14	1881	51	1876	1.52	2003
1	02	43	29	0.08	0.2	71	1876	15	1918	-1	1899	52	1876	1.44	1979
1	03	43	29	0.09	0.1	68	2004	10	1879	-3	1877	52	2000	1.87	1914
					. . .				. . .						
12	31	44	29	0.08	0.1	70	1965	12	1917	-13	1880	52	1884	1.68	1975

Source: National Weather Service.
The columns of these data are as follows.
(A) Month and day of the year.
(B) Normal maximum and minimum temperature for that day.
(C) Normal precipitation/snow.
(D) Record maximum temperature and year.
(E) Lowest recorded maximum and year.
(F) Record minimum and year.
(G) Highest recorded minimum and year.
(H) Highest recorded precipitation and year.

$p = 0.5$. That is, record high temperatures are much more likely to appear in more recent years than record cold temperatures.

a. Fit a logistic regression to the data of Table 9.5 where the binary values' response is whether or not the highest recorded temperatures occurred before or after the lowest recorded temperatures. For explanatory variables we might use the normal highs and lows for that day of the year. The interpretation of the model is to see whether record highs or lows are more recently occurring in warmer or colder times of the year. Do influential observations occur randomly or are these concentrated at certain times of the year?

b. Extremes in temperature may not be representative of overall climate. The data in Table 9.5 includes the lowest high and the highest low along with the corresponding record years. The lowest high is indicative of a cooler temperature all day long, rather than an extreme recorded at just one brief time during the day. Similarly, a highest low indicates an overall warm day. Does logistic regression tell us about the appearances of low highs and high lows in the historical record? Do these values tell the same story as in part (a)?

10 Poisson Regression

The Poisson[1] distribution is the approximation to the binomial model when the N parameter is large and the p parameter is small. This is probably the most important discrete distribution for public health. Many individuals are at risk for events very unlikely to occur to any one of them. Shark attacks, lottery winners, and lightning strikes are all good examples. So is the incidence of cancer, industrial injuries, surgical complications, and the births of twins.

10.1 Lottery Winners

Let us consider the example of people winning the lottery in several different towns in the New Haven area. The data is given in Table 10.1. There are a large number of people playing, many tickets are sold, but the probability of winning remains very small. Yet, as the advertisements point out, some people do win. In a town with a population of a few thousand, how can we develop mathematical models to describe the numbers of winners? What about characteristics of different towns: Do rural or urban settings have more winners? Do towns with higher property taxes have a different number of winners? How do we take into account the different population sizes of the various towns? We show how to answer some of these questions and leave the remainder for the reader to complete in the exercise of Section 10.6.4.

10.2 Poisson Distribution Basics

Recall the binomial experiment described in Section 2.1. A simple experiment is repeated N times, and each independent outcome occurs as success with probability p or failure with probability $1 - p$. The Poisson distribution is an approximation to the binomial model where N is large and p is small. In our lottery example, there are many lottery players and many tickets are sold, but a very small chance any one ticket wins a major prize.

---

[1] Siméon-Denis Poisson, French physicist and mathematician (1781–1840), published this statistical distribution in 1838. Poisson is the French word for fish.

Table 10.1 The number of lottery winners in towns near New Haven. Columns are town name; number of lottery winners; population (in thousands); area in square miles; property tax mill rate; and number of library books per student.

Town	Winners	Pop.	Area	Mill	Books
Ansonia	6	17.9	6.2	28.9	16.4
Branford	11	28.0	27.9	22.6	18.0
Cheshire	6	26.2	33.0	27.1	21.0
Clinton	2	12.8	17.2	27.9	20.5
Derby	6	12.0	5.3	29.6	14.8
East Haven	9	26.5	12.6	37.1	13.5
Guilford	6	20.3	47.7	28.6	30.9
Hamden	9	52.0	33.0	34.1	17.4
Madison	5	16.0	36.3	22.3	24.2
Milford	10	49.5	23.5	30.8	19.7
N. Branford	2	13.1	26.8	26.9	14.0
North Haven	12	21.6	21.0	23.4	23.2
Old Saybrook	1	9.3	18.3	15.3	23.4
Orange	9	12.5	17.6	23.8	29.7
Oxford	3	9.1	33.0	29.0	15.3
Seymour	1	14.5	14.7	40.5	18.7
Shelton	7	36.0	31.4	21.6	17.3
Trumbull	14	33.0	23.5	24.1	21.6
West Haven	12	54.0	10.6	41.4	17.2
Woodbridge	1	8.0	19.3	28.4	43.0

Sources: New Haven Register, August 17, 1995, and US Census data.

> The Poisson distribution is the approximation
> to the binomial for large N and small p.

It is hard to say exactly where the approximation takes over. Larger N and smaller p make it better, but there are no quick rules about when the Poisson is to be preferred to the binomial model. If it was essential we get the right value, then we should not cut any corners in getting it correct and use the binomial distribution. On the other hand, finding factorials of really large numbers in order to calculate the binomial probability may quickly dissuade us from using it. Exercise 10.1 asks the reader to calculate some probabilities and note how well the approximation works for a simple example.

The Poisson model assumes the binomial mean Np is fixed and moderate. We don't want to talk about a setting where Np is small so there are too few rare events expected. Similarly, if Np is large, then we would do better to use the normal approximation to the binomial model.

Recall from (2.3), the variance of the binomial distribution is equal to $Np(1 - p)$. When p is very close to 0, then $1 - p$ is very close to 1 and can be ignored in the variance. This makes the variance very close to the value Np, or the same as the mean. So, when N is large and p is small, we see the mean and the variance are very close in value.

> In the Poisson distribution, the mean and variance are equal in value.

In the Poisson distribution, we do not talk about the N and p parts separately. Instead we refer to the distribution by its mean, which we denote using the Greek letter lambda, λ. The value of λ can be any positive number, and it does not need to be an integer. The value of λ is both the mean and the variance, as we just pointed out.

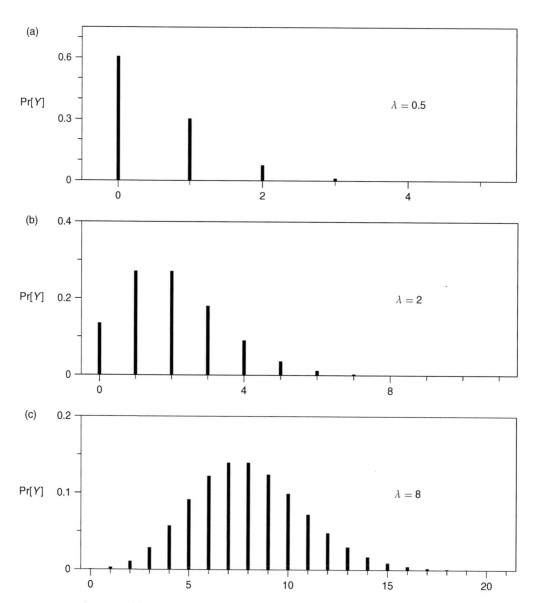

Figure 10.1 The Poisson distribution illustrated for values of λ equal to (a) 0.5, (b) 2, and (c) 8.

As with the binomial distribution, the outcome must be a nonnegative integer number of events. The range of the Poisson distribution is infinite because the N part of the binomial is considered to be very large.

In a Poisson distribution with mean λ, the probability of j events (for any value of $j = 0, 1, 2, \ldots$) is equal to

$$\Pr[\, j \text{ events}\,] = e^{-\lambda}\lambda^{j}/j!\,. \tag{10.1}$$

We do not need to know this formula in order to use the Poisson distribution or fit models to it. The formula is useful to illustrate the shape of the distribution. Examples of the Poisson distribution are given in Fig. 10.1 for values of λ equal to 0.5, 2, and 8.

When the Poisson mean λ is equal to 0.5, we see in Fig. 10.1 (a) that most of the probability is concentrated at 0 and 1 events, and larger values are unlikely to occur. Even though the distribution continues on to the right forever, these probabilities quickly become very small. When λ is increased to 2, Fig. 10.1 (b) shows the variance as well as the mean have increased. The range of likely values has increased to between 0 and 5, and values larger than 7 should rarely appear. When $\lambda = 8$, Fig. 10.1 (c) shows the Poisson is starting to look much like a normal distribution.

> The Poisson distribution with a large mean is approximately normal.

10.3   Statistics in the News: Terror Attacks

Terror attacks are a sad fact of life, but fortunately these have been decreasing in frequency. Figure 10.2 (a) shows the total numbers of casualties in Western Europe through 2014. The figure shows the total numbers of deaths fluctuated widely by year but greatly decreased in recent years. The value for 1993 is missing. The attacks are classified as Islamic-based or not. Very few of these have Islamic connections.

Figure 10.2 (b) concentrates on only the most recent years and tells a completely different story. Recent years show an increase in terrorism deaths and the majority of these are jihadist but these rates are far below the number of deaths experienced in the 1970s and 1980s.

Many innocent people are at risk but the probability of being involved is very small. The values for each year are an example of the Poisson distribution. In years with large values, there is also a large amount of variability, just as we would expect from the Poisson model.

The decreasing trend is probably due to increased vigilance by police, as well as the public. Is there a similar trend of a greater or fewer number of deaths per attack? We would need a separate graph of the numbers of attacks each year to estimate this rate.

Are the counts independent from one year to the next? There are copy-cat attacks, but then again, authorities are on alert following one event for another similar act. Counts in adjacent years of a *time series* such as this should be more highly correlated than those more distant in time. Such data is often said to be *autocorrelated*, meaning

(a)

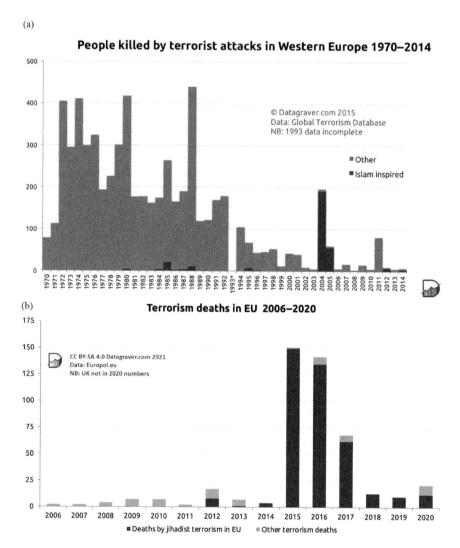

Figure 10.2 History of terror attacks.
Source: Datagraver.

the correlation between observations at two points falls off with the time difference between them. Autocorrelated time series data, usually with calendar effects, often appears in studies of economic activity in which events in one time period have bearing on the nearby periods but little effect years later.

10.4   Regression Models for Poisson Data

In Poisson regression, we model λ, the mean number of events. The aim is to see how λ varies with additional covariate information available in the data. Are there more lottery winners, for example, in towns with larger areas?

We should avoid the temptation to fit a model of the form

$$\lambda = \alpha + \beta_1 \text{ Area} + \beta_2 \text{ Population}.$$

For some values of the area and population, this might result in a negative number but we must always have $\lambda > 0$. Instead, we need to use a link function.

Just as we used a link function in Chapter 8 for logistic regression, we need a way to link the mean of the distribution with the linear combination of explanatory covariates. The specific link used in Poisson regression is the log function. (The logarithm, as elsewhere in this book, is to the base e $= 2.718\ldots$).

In Poisson regression, we fit models of the form

$$\log(\lambda) = \alpha + \beta_1 x_1 + \beta_2 x_2 + \cdots$$

for explanatory variables x_1, x_2, $\ldots$.

Equivalently,

$$\lambda = \exp(\alpha + \beta_1 x_1 + \beta_2 x_2 + \cdots),$$

so the estimated values of λ can never be negative, regardless of the values of the xs or the estimated parameters α and the βs.

A program to fit a Poisson regression model to the lottery data is given in Output 10.1. We use glm and include the family = to specify the distribution using a syntax similar to the way we specified logistic regression in the previous chapter.

Output 10.1 A program to fit a Poisson regression model to the lottery data.

```
> lottery <- read.table(file = "lottery.txt", header = TRUE)
> lottery[1:3,]                    #  echo some of the data
        town winners  pop area mill books
1  Ansonia        6 17.9  6.2 28.9  16.4
2 Branford       11 28.0 27.9 22.6  18.0
3 Cheshire        6 26.2 33.0 27.1  21.0
> lot.Poi <- glm(winners ~ pop + area + mill + books,
+                data = lottery, family = poisson)
> summary(lot.Poi)               # estimated parameters, significance

            .    .    .    .

Coefficients:
              Estimate Std. Error z value Pr(>|z|)
(Intercept)  2.3173603  0.6705173   3.456 0.000548 ***
pop          0.0338097  0.0072435   4.668 3.05e-06 ***
area        -0.0135763  0.0103170  -1.316 0.188205
mill        -0.0363749  0.0174699  -2.082 0.037329 *
books        0.0006178  0.0171971   0.036 0.971343

            .    .    .    .
```

The `glm` statement in Output 10.1 fits models for `winners` as a Poisson count. The `family = poisson` option specifies the response variable (`winners`) has a Poisson distribution. The log of the mean number of winners is linear in the covariates area and population. The log is the default link in Poisson regression and does not need to be specified in the `glm` statement.

The `glm` statement in Output 10.1 specifies the model

$$\log(\lambda_i) = \alpha + \beta_1\, \mathtt{pop}_i + \beta_2\, \mathtt{area}_i \beta_3\, \mathtt{mill}_i + \beta_4\, \mathtt{books}_i, \qquad (10.2)$$

where λ_i is the mean number of lottery winners we expect in the ith town.

A portion of the output is given in Output 10.1. The summary statement produces output including parameter estimates, standard errors, and tests of their statistical significance. This output contains the fitted parameters for α, and the βs. Each of these estimated parameters is accompanied by its estimated standard error. The z-value statistic is the ratio of the parameter estimate divided by its estimated standard error. Under the null hypothesis that the underlying (population) parameter value is zero, this statistic behaves as standard normal. The p-value for this test is given in the last column of the table.

In this output, we can see town population is very important in explaining the mean number of lottery winners in the various towns. The town's mill rate also has some explanatory value in this model. The mill rate is the tax paid on real estate and is explained in Section 10.6.4.

A number of diagnostics are available to us through `glm`. Output 10.2 illustrates how to obtain these in **R**, and Fig. 10.3 presents two useful plots. The estimated

---

Output 10.2 Poisson regression model diagnostics in the lottery data.

```
> inf <- influence(lot.Poi)      # residuals, hat matrix, dfbeta
>
> lam.hat <- fitted(lot.Poi)     # estimated Poisson means, lambda
> plot(lam.hat, inf$dev.res,     # plot deviance residuals
+      xlab = "Fitted values", ylab = "Deviance residuals",
+      cex.lab = 1.25)
> lines(c(2,14), c(0,0))         # add x-axis
> br <- match(sort(inf$dev.res)[1], inf$dev.res) # identify large residual
> text(lam.hat[br], inf$dev.res[br], pos = 2,
+      labels = lottery$town[br])


> # Plot hat diagonals and identify two influential towns
> plot(lam.hat, inf$hat,         # hat matrix diagonal
+      xlab = "Fitted values", ylab = "Hat diagonals",
+      cex.lab = 1.25)
> tb <- match( -sort(-inf$hat)[1:2], inf$hat) # identify 2 biggest
> text(lam.hat[tb], inf$hat[tb], pos = c(4,2),
+      labels = lottery$town[tb], cex = 1.15)
```

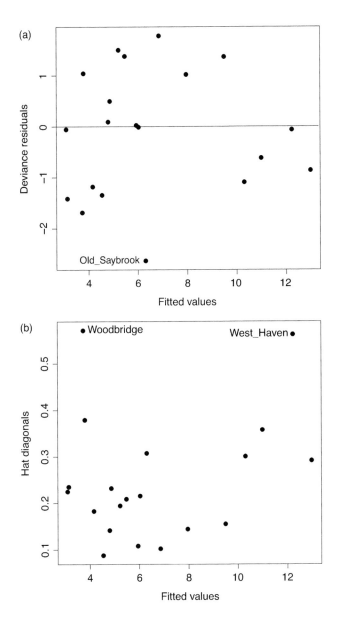

Figure 10.3 Diagnostics for Poisson regression on lottery data, produced by the code in Output 10.2.

mean number of winners for each of the towns $\hat{\lambda}_i$ are obtained from the `fitted()` program. The `influence` program produces two types of residuals, and a variety of useful diagnostic measures including the hat diagonal and dfbeta's for the estimated regression coefficients.

The Pearson residual is obtained as `$pear.res` from the `influence` program. These are defined

$$\text{Pearson residual}_i = (\texttt{winners}_i - \hat{\lambda}_i) \Big/ \sqrt{\hat{\lambda}_i},$$

where the denominator is chosen because the mean is equal to the variance in the Poisson distribution. The sum of squared Pearson residuals is the familiar chi-squared statistic which is useful in testing overall fit of the model in a setting where all estimated means are large.

The *deviance* is another statistic behaving similarly to the chi-squared statistic. In Poisson regression, the estimated values of the βs are found by minimizing the deviance, rather than through least squares as is the case in linear regression. The deviance statistic for Poisson regression is

$$\text{Deviance} = \sum_i (\texttt{winners}_i - \hat{\lambda}_i) + \texttt{winners}_i \, \log(\hat{\lambda}_i / \texttt{winners}_i),$$

where $\texttt{winners}_i$ is the observed Poisson count in the i-th town.

Similarly, the deviance residual is defined as

$$\text{Deviance residual} = \pm\sqrt{(\texttt{winners}_i - \hat{\lambda}_i) + \texttt{winners}_i \, \log(\hat{\lambda}_i / \texttt{winners}_i)},$$

where the $\pm$ is determined by whether the number of winners is larger than or less than the estimated number $\hat{\lambda}_i$ for the ith town.

The deviance residuals are plotted in Fig. 10.3 (a) and demonstrate a reasonable overall fit to the model. One moderate outlier is identified. The Pearson residuals and the deviance residuals usually have very nearly the same numerical values.

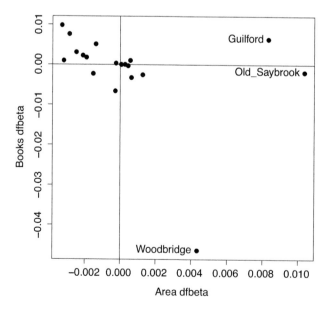

Figure 10.4 Lottery data dfbetas for area and books.

The hat diagonals are also available to identify observations with high influence. In Output 10.2, we see these are obtained using $hat from the influence() program. The hat values are plotted in Fig. 10.3 (b) and two influential towns are identified.

More specific than the hat diagnostic are individual dfbeta's for each regression coefficient. As with linear regresson, the dfbeta measures how much an estimated regression coefficient changes when each observation is jackknifed (omitted) and the model is refitted.

Figure 10.4 plots the dfbetas for area and number of books in the lottery data. This figure shows influential observations along separate axes. Three influential towns are identified: Old Saybrook and Woodbridge have very small areas, and Guilford has a large number of books per student. Old Saybrook and Woodbridge were also identified as unusual in Fig. 10.3.

10.5   The Offset

Suppose we want to model the mean number of lottery winners as proportional to the town's population. In a town with twice the population, we should expect to see twice the number of lottery winners, all other things remaining equal. In vital rates, as another example, we want to talk about the number of cases of mortality and morbidity relative to the population at risk. How do we do this? Before we can answer this question, we need to describe what it means to be *proportional to*.

If population was the only thing that mattered in describing the expected number of lottery winners λ_i in the ith town then we would have the model

$$\lambda_i = C \times \text{Population}_i,$$

where C has the same value for all towns, like a regression coefficient. So if the population doubles, the mean number of lottery winners (λ) also doubles.

Then the corresponding log-link gives the model

$$\log(\lambda_i) = \log(C) + \log(\text{Population}_i).$$

This last equation illustrates the problem in fitting a *proportional to* model. We need to estimate C, but there is no regression coefficient to be estimated for the $\log(\text{Population}_i)$ term. More accurately, the regression coefficient in front of

$$\log(\text{Population}_i)$$

is always equal to 1.

If we want to include covariates such as area and mill rate in our model but still keep the mean number of lottery winners proportional to the population, then we might fit a model of the form

$$\lambda_i = C \times \text{Population}_i \times \exp(\beta_1 \text{Area}_i + \beta_2 \text{Mill}_i)$$

so

$$\log(\lambda_i) = \log(C) + \log(\text{Population}_i) + \beta_1 \text{Area}_i + \beta_2 \text{Mill}_i. \qquad (10.3)$$

Again we see the term $\log(\text{Population}_i)$ is not associated with any estimated regression coefficient. The intercept is the same as $\log(C)$, so this is not an issue. The regression coefficients β_1, and β_2 can be estimated using the Poisson regression methods we have already described. Together this gives us model (10.3) adjusting for the effects of the covariates (area and mill rate) and also specifies the mean number of lottery winners proportional to the population size.

We have just illustrated the model we need to fit in order to produce estimates based on a "proportional to" model. In this case we fit a model similar to a Poisson regression, but the $\log(\text{Population})$ term in model (10.3) doesn't have a regression coefficient. Or, more correctly, $\log(\text{Population})$ has a regression coefficient identically equal to 1. Such a term can be added to the model using the offset in glm.

Output 10.3 Program to illustrate offset in Poisson regression.

```
> logPop <- log(lottery$pop)     # create offset variate
>
> glm(winners ~ logPop + area + mill,
+     family = poisson, data = lottery)

Call:  glm(formula = winners ~ logPop + area + mill, family = poisson,
       data = lottery)

Coefficients:
(Intercept)         logPop           area           mill
    0.21337        0.99095       -0.01741       -0.03633

Degrees of Freedom: 19 Total (i.e. Null);  16 Residual
Null Deviance:      53.92
Residual Deviance: 21.64          AIC: 99.51
>
> glm(winners ~ area + mill,
+     offset = logPop,
+     family = poisson, data = lottery)

Call:  glm(formula = winners ~ area + mill, family = poisson, data = lottery,
       offset = logPop)

Coefficients:
(Intercept)           area           mill
    0.20091       -0.01760       -0.03677

Degrees of Freedom: 19 Total (i.e. Null);  17 Residual
Null Deviance:      29
Residual Deviance: 21.64          AIC: 97.51
```

An example of the use of an `offset` is given in Output 10.3. We begin by creating a new variable (`logPop`) equal to the logarithm of the town's population. When we use this variable in a regression, the estimated coefficient is 0.99095, or almost 1, suggesting the use of an offset. The deviance for this model is 21.64.

The second model fitted in Output 10.3 uses the offset option. The log population does not appear in the list of fitted regression coefficients. The model deviance is 21.64, the same as in the model including log population as a covariate in the model. Similarly, there is no test of statistical significance for the log population.

In the case of the lottery data, an offset is not only appropriate, but is suggested by the data analysis as well. The deviance is unchanged when we estimate a regression coefficient or force it into the model with a coefficient of 1. The estimated coefficient is almost exactly equal to 1. The resulting model has an intuitive interpretation, namely the number of lottery winners is proportional to the town's population with smaller adjustments for other covariates.

10.6 Exercises

10.1 In a Poisson distribution with a mean of 1, find the probability of two or fewer events. In a binomial experiment with $N = 4$ and $p = 1/4$, what is the probability of two or fewer events? In a binomial experiment with $N = 8$ and $p = 1/8$, what is the probability of two or fewer events? What is the mean for both of these binomial experiments? What are the variances? Do the variances in these two binomial models become closer to the means as N gets larger and p becomes smaller? Do the probabilities of two or fewer events get closer to the Poisson approximation?

10.2 In Output 10.3, we used log population as an offset where the population is measured as thousands of persons. What happens if we measure population in counts of individual people? Does it matter which definition we use? Run the program in Output 10.3 using both definitions and note the differences in the output. Can you explain the differences in the outputs?

10.6.1 Coronary Bypass Mortality, Revisited

Reexamine the mortality data in Section 5.7.3 using Poisson regression. Specifically, consider the number of in-hospital deaths as a Poisson-distributed outcome. Why is the Poisson distribution a reasonable assumption? Do the residuals of the fitted regression model correspond to the indications of higher and lower death rates given by the last column of Table 5.3?

10.6.2 Cases of Mental Illness

A historical survey of cases of mental illness (who were then called *lunatics*) in Massachusetts in the 1850s is presented in Table 10.2. For each of the 14 counties, we have the number of patients, the distance to the nearest mental health center, the

Table 10.2 Number of cases of mental illness in Massachusetts by county in 1854.

County	Cases	Distance to mental health center	Population in 1000s	Population density	Percentage cared for at home
Berkshire	119	97	26.656	56	77
Franklin	84	62	22.260	45	81
Hampshire	94	54	23.312	72	75
Hampden	105	52	18.900	94	69
Worcester	351	20	82.836	98	64
Middlesex	357	14	66.759	231	47
Essex	377	10	95.004	3252	47
Suffolk	458	4	123.202	3042	6
Norfolk	241	14	62.901	235	49
Bristol	158	14	29.704	151	60
Plymouth	139	16	32.526	91	68
Barnstable	78	44	16.692	93	76
Nantucket	12	77	1.740	179	25
Dukes	19	52	7.524	46	79

Available in **R** as `lunatics` in the BaM library.

population (in thousands), the population density (per square mile), and the percentage of patients cared for at home.

The counties have very different characteristics: Suffolk County includes Boston; Duke County (Martha's Vineyard) and Nantucket are islands; and Berkshire County is farthest from Boston, in the western part of the state. The great population differences argue for using the logarithm of population rather than the original population values.

Show the number of cases varies with either population, or log population, as we would expect. Why is the population density such a good explanatory variable in this data set? Does the distance to a mental health center explain the number of cases or does it explain the number of diagnosed cases? Does the reciprocal distance provide a better interpretation or offer better explanatory value? In other words, is there evidence of undiagnosed or missing cases?

In a separate analysis using regression methods, does the rate of home treatment vary with population density or distance to a center? Why is this the case?

10.6.3   Airlines Bump Passengers

Running an airline is an expensive business, and unsold seats cut into profits. Airlines have long known each flight will have a small number of passengers with reservations who do not show up. To decrease the chances of lost revenue, the airlines will usually sell more seats than exist. If too many passengers show up, the airlines will need to bump passengers to a later flight, first asking for volunteers by offering successively higher incentives (such as cash or vouchers for future flights and hotels) and finally involuntary measures. This, of course, creates a lot of bad feelings and publicity.

Involuntary removals from flights are declining

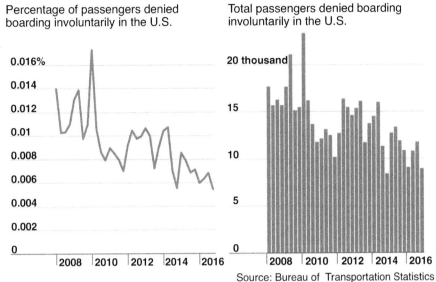

Percentage of passengers denied boarding involuntarily in the U.S.

Total passengers denied boarding involuntarily in the U.S.

Source: Bureau of Transportation Statistics

Figure 10.5 Statistics on airline bumping of passengers.

Anxious passengers have taken to making several reservations under fictitious names in order to ensure the real passengers are unlikely to be bumped.

Why do you think a Poisson distribution would be appropriate to model the number of no-shows on a flight? What assumptions do you consider? Each airline has its own formula, but the probability of being bumped is a small fraction of 1%, according to Fig. 10.5. What information would you need to estimate the number of no-shows on future flights? Would flights with a large percentage of business travelers have a different rate than flights to vacation destinations? Would the rate for large planes to big cities differ from smaller regional flights with fewer seats? Explain why or why not you think this may be the case.

Compare the two graphics of the number of passengers who were bumped. Both the percent and number of passengers is decreasing. Would it also be useful to know how many passengers flew in each time period?

In this exercise, suppose an airline routinely reserves up to 190 passengers for a flight with only 185 physical seats. That is, they are counting on 5 or more no-shows. From experience, the airline expects a small percentage of those passengers to fail to show up at the time of the flight. Estimate the Poisson parameter λ for the number of no-shows out of 190 potential passengers on this flight so there is at most a 0.1% probability at least one passenger will be bumped.

Hint: Use

```
sum(dpois(0 : 4, lambda = ...  ))
```

in **R** to compute the Poisson probability of 4 or fewer no-shows on this flight for a specified value of lambda. By trial and error, find the value of λ so this probability is smaller than 0.001.

Similarly, how many seats can the airline sell and be 99% certain nobody will be bumped?

10.6.4   Lottery Winners

Table 10.1 lists the number of lottery winners in several towns near New Haven, Connecticut. The columns in this table are town name; the number of lottery winners (the response or Y variable); the town's area in square miles; mill rate; and the number of library books per student.

The mill rate is the tax rate paid per $1000 value of real estate. Industrial properties generally pay a higher rate than residential ones. Undeveloped or vacant land also pays a lower rate. The mill rate is a surrogate for property values: lower rates usually appear in towns with higher property values. The mill rate may also reflect the services a town provides. A town with volunteer firefighters, for example, will tend to have a lower mill rate than a town with a paid fire-fighting force. Similarly, a town with a lot of open space or farmland will have fewer public services than a more urban town. However, the rural town will also have fewer homes and businesses to generate other tax revenue. You can create a new explanatory variable measuring population density (population divided by area). Density is a measure of urban or rural character of a town.

Using your final model, estimate the number of lottery winners expected in the city of New Haven with a population of 126,000, an area of 21.1 square miles, and a mill rate of 37.0. What about the town of Durham with 6000 people, 23.3 square miles, and a mill rate of 26.4? Are these appropriate uses of your model? Explain.

Are some towns luckier than others? Is the number of winners proportional to the population? Should it be? What can you say about the intercept, on a log scale? What other covariate values might be useful to you? Is the Poisson distribution appropriate for this example? Why?

10.6.5   Species on the Galápagos Islands

Follow Charles Darwin to the Galápagos Islands! These islands are hundreds of miles from the nearest continent. Their flora and fauna are the subject of many scientific studies. The summary of one such survey is given in Table 10.3. The data variables are island name, the number of plant species (the dependent variable), area in square kilometers, distance to nearest neighboring island, distance to Santa Cruz (the second largest island, near the center of the archipelago), and the number of species on the nearest neighboring island.

Use the Poisson distribution to model the number of species on each of these islands. Larger islands support a larger diversity of life forms. Isabela is so much

Table 10.3 Diversity of plant species on each of the Galápagos Islands.

Island	Species observed	Area in km^2	Elevation in m	Distance (km) To nearest neighbor	Distance (km) To Santa Cruz	Species on adjacent island
Baltra	58	25.09	346	0.6	0.6	44
Bartolomé	31	1.24	109	0.6	26.3	237
Caldwell	3	0.21	114	2.8	58.7	5
⋮						
Wolf	21	2.85	253	34.1	254.7	10

Available in **R** as `gala` in the `faraway` library.

larger than all the other islands that it exerts a high amount of leverage. You might want to create a separate indicator for Isabela. Create new variables such as products (interactions) and ratios of variables you can interpret. Are there outliers in the data? Are small islands similar to each other or very different from each other? What about the larger islands?

Is the Poisson model appropriate for this data? You can sometimes use the Poisson distribution for settings where there is no underlying binomial model to be approximated: that is, where there is no N or p. Another use of the Poisson model without an underlying binomial model appears in Exercise 10.6.8.

Is there an evolutionary advantage to species on an island with a larger diversity of lifeforms? We might see this if the islands with large estimated numbers of species appear to have too many species and, similarly, if those with small estimated numbers would tend to have fewer than expected. The result would be both the upper and lower tails of the Poisson distribution extend out further than we would expect. Does this help explain some of the outliers in the data? Are there other explanations for these outliers? Should all species be treated equally, for example?

10.6.6   Sports Statistics: Pro Bowl Appearances

Football is a game of strength and speed. Running with the ball is appropriately called *rushing*. The total career distances covered by the most accomplished players at the time of the source publication[2] are listed in Table 10.4. Most of the players listed had retired. The men whose names are listed as active were still playing. The article accompanying this table concentrates on Fred Taylor, who was close to having rushed 10,000 career yards but had not yet appeared in a Pro Bowl.

The Pro Bowl is played at the end of the regular season by players who are judged to be the best individual players, regardless of their regular team. The game itself is not taken as seriously as regular season games because these are players who have

---

[2] www.nytimes.com/2007/11/02/sports/football/02taylor.html.

Table 10.4 Pro Bowl appearances by running backs.

Name	Active?	Career Yards	Pro Bowls
Emmit Smith	N	18,355	8
Walter Payton	N	16,726	9
Barry Sanders	N	15,269	10
Curtis Martin	N	14,101	5
Jerome Bettis	N	13,662	6
Eric Dickerson	N	13,259	5
Tony Dorsett	N	12,739	4
Jim Brown	N	12,312	9
Marshall Faulk	N	12,279	7
Marcus Allen	N	12,243	6
Franco Harris	N	12,120	8
Thurman Harris	N	12,074	5
John Riggins	N	11,352	1
Corey Dillon	N	11,241	4
O.J. Simpson	N	11,236	5
Edgerrin James	Y	10,988	3
Ricky Watters	N	10,643	5
Tiki Barber	N	10,449	3
Eddie George	N	10,441	4
Ottis Anderson	N	10,273	2
Fred Taylor	Y	9,933	0
LaDainian Tomlinson	Y	9,793	4
Warrick Dunn	Y	9,753	3
Earl Campbell	Y	9,407	5
Shaun Alexander	Y	9,173	3

Reported by the *New York Times*, November 2, 2007.

likely never practiced together. There is a lot of friendly camaraderie. The rules are relaxed so the play is not nearly as competitive. Rather, it is considered a great honor to be chosen to play. Table 10.4 lists the players with the top 25 rushing records and includes the number of Pro Bowl appearances of each.

Use Poisson regression to show larger numbers of rushing yards are associated with a larger number of career Pro Bowl appearances. Create an indicator variable for active versus retired status and include this in your model. Is there a significant interaction between this indicator and total rushing yards? How do you interpret this finding? Does Fred Taylor appear to be an outlier, never having been chosen to play in the Pro Bowl? Compare his residual with that of John Riggins, for example, who had only one Pro Bowl appearance. Are there other outliers in these data worth noting? Can you identify players whose records were overrated, resulting in too many Pro Bowl appearances?

A small number of players appear to have much stronger rushing records than the rest. Try transforming the rushing yards variable by log or square root to remove the influence these players have on the fitted model. Does this model result in a better fit?

Say something about the overall fit of the model. Does this appear to be a valid use of the Poisson model? Can you justify the use of the model in this case? Is the use of the Poisson model any less valid than its use in the species data of Exercise 10.6.5?

10.6.7 Cancer Rates in Japan

Vital rates are important for many reasons and are collected by government agencies. We saw an example of this in Section 3.5.6. This exercise represents another example of official mortality data. The data of Table 10.5 summarizes the number of men in Japan who died of cancer of the testis in 1946–70 by five-year intervals. The populations are given in thousands. The rows are the ages given in five-year groups. Missing data are indicated by asterisks and these should be omitted in any examination of these data.

Output 10.4 gives **R** code to read, reformat, and perform Poisson regression on these data. The ages are converted to categories with values $1, 2, \ldots, 18$, and the five time periods are similarly converted. The as.factor program in glm converts age and period categories into a series of indicator variables. The first of these is omitted to avoid multicolinearity. (See Section 6.1 for more on this.)

Table 10.5 Deaths in Japan due to cancer of the testis by age, year, and population (in thousands). The values indicated by '*' are missing.

Age	1947–49 Pop.	Deaths	1951–55 Pop.	Deaths	1956–60 Pop.	Deaths	1961–65 Pop.	Deaths	1966–70 Pop.	Deaths
0	15,501	17	26,914	51	21,027	65	20,246	69	21,596	74
5	14,236	*	25,380	6	26,613	7	20,885	8	20,051	7
10	13,270	*	23,492	3	25,324	3	26,540	7	20,718	11
15	12,658	2	21,881	6	23,211	15	24,931	25	26,182	39
20	10,696	5	20,402	27	21,263	39	22,228	56	24,033	83
25	7,563	5	17,242	40	19,994	58	20,606	97	21,805	125
30	7,074	7	12,609	18	17,128	54	19,864	77	20,750	129
35	7,038	10	11,712	13	12,476	36	17,001	70	19,890	101
40	6,418	9	11,478	26	11,450	32	12,275	29	16,794	67
45	5,981	7	10,274	16	11,157	26	11,147	34	11,962	37
50	4,944	7	9,325	16	9,828	27	10,705	27	10,741	29
55	3,994	7	7,562	17	8,718	19	9,206	32	10,086	39
60	3,098	6	5,902	13	6,796	21	7,869	21	8,399	31
65	2,317	4	4,244	12	4,911	26	5,728	29	6,715	34
70	1,513	7	2,845	17	3,197	22	3,737	25	4,448	33
75	688	5	1,587	9	1,812	10	2,061	25	2,482	31
80	264	2	583	6	787	6	904	14	1,068	9
85	73	2	179	2	246	3	335	3	419	3

Public domain: *Journal of the National Cancer Institute*, Oxford University Press. See also Lee *et al.* (1973) and Andrews and Herzberg (1985, pp. 233–5).

Is the Poisson distribution appropriate for this data? Why? Fit a model with effects for year periods and ages. Look at the residuals. Plot the estimated cohort and age effects to show any general trends. Are there any trends over the years?

A *cohort* is the same group of men appearing several times in this table. Five years later, the men from one age/year group are five years older and will appear again in the next age/year group. The cohort runs diagonally from upper left to lower right. The cohort category is also given in Output 10.4.

Output 10.4 Read, reformat, and fit the Japanese cancer data.

```
> canc <- read.table(file = "cancer.txt", header = T)
> canc[1:3, ]                         # echo a few rows
  age pop47 d47 pop51 d51 pop56 d56 pop61 d61 pop66 d66
1   0 15501  17 26914  51 21027  65 20246  69 21596  74
2   5 14236  NA 25380   6 26613   7 20885   8 20051   7
3  10 13270  NA 23492   3 25324   3 26540   7 20718  11
> age    <- rep(1:18, 5)                    # age category
> pop <- c(canc$pop47, canc$pop51, canc$pop56, canc$pop61, canc$pop66)
> death <- c(canc$d47, canc$d51, canc$d56, canc$d61, canc$d66)
> period <- rep(1:5, each = 18)      # period categories
> cohort <- age  - period
> cohort <- cohort - min(cohort) +1 # categories start at 1
> cancer <- cbind(death, pop, age , period, cohort)
> cancer <- data.frame(cancer)
> cancer                             # reformatted
  death    pop age period cohort
1    17  15501   1      1      5
2    NA  14236   2      1      6
3    NA  13270   3      1      7
4     2  12658   4      1      8
```

                    .   .   .

```
> glm(death ~ as.factor(age) + as.factor(cohort),
+       offset = log(pop),
+       family = poisson, data = cancer)

Call:  glm(formula = death ~ as.factor(age) + as.factor(cohort),
        family = poisson,  data = cancer, offset = log(pop))

Coefficients:
          (Intercept)      as.factor(age)2      as.factor(age)3
             -5.67620             -2.02251             -1.91019
      as.factor(age)4      as.factor(age)5      as.factor(age)6
             -0.26270              1.14727              2.06341
```

                    .   .   .

Try to fit a model including the three separate effects of age, period, and cohort. What happens? Can you explain this problem? Reread the discussion of multicolinearity in Section 6.1 and describe the difficulty with the *age, period, cohort model.*

10.6.8   Tourette's Syndrome

In an experiment conducted at the Yale Child Study Center, van Wattum *et al.* (2000) studied the effects of naloxone on patients diagnosed with Tourette's syndrome. Patients with Tourette's syndrome suffer from frequent involuntary twitches (motor) or verbal (phonic) outbursts. Naloxone is usually administered to counteract the effects of narcotic drug overdoses. Naloxone (also known as NARCAN and EVZIO) is used for other medical treatments, and its effects are well studied. In this experiment, it was thought naloxone inhibits certain receptors in the brain and perhaps small amounts could reduce the symptoms of Tourette's.

Fourteen patients were each given one of three different doses of naloxone, and their behaviors were recorded during three one-hour periods of observation. Motor and phonic tics were counted separately for each of the three time periods. The data for the patients, naloxone dose, and tics for each of the three time periods is given in Table 10.6.

It is not clear whether we should be separately modeling the motor and phonic tics. Perhaps the sum of these two measures is more appropriate. As with the species example in Section 10.6.5, there is no underlying binomial experiment we can refer to, so there are no N or p parameters. Instead, we might think of a subject's brain

Table 10.6 Motor and phonic tics in Tourette's patients treated with naloxone during three one-hour time periods.

Patient number	Naloxone dose (mcg)	Period I		Period II		Period III	
		Motor	Phonic	Motor	Phonic	Motor	Phonic
1	300	90	45	86	51	106	57
2	30	75	0	243	0	152	0
3	30	58	0	9	0	22	0
4	30	13	0	6	0	12	0
5	30	13	0	16	0	29	0
6	300	150	0	161	0	121	0
7	30	49	1	16	0	29	1
8	30	27	0	28	0	24	0
9	0	25	7	9	0	4	4
10	0	13	2	14	17	14	18
11	300	51	0	42	0	43	0
12	300	35	16	28	33	49	20
13	300	19	9	8	15	12	30
14	30	8	6	18	13	8	22

Source: van Wattum *et al.* (2000).

sending and receiving a great many signals, and a small fraction of these are either misinterpreted or sent incorrectly.

The three separate periods were part of the experiment to see if the number of tics would change as the subject became acclimatized to the investigators and their settings. The investigators thought a subject in unfamiliar surroundings would be more self-conscious and the number of tics would decrease. Similarly, after the subjects relaxed on their second or third visits, perhaps their tics might resume. Do you see evidence of a period effect in the numbers of either the motor or verbal tics? How can you justify modeling the log mean for this data?

Examine the two separate doses and compare the tic rates with those of the control. Is there any difference in these rates? Include a period effect in your model. Is the naloxone effect larger or smaller than the period effect?

11 Survival Analysis

Survival data, despite its name, is concerned with the time to an event, not just the death of the subject. The event could be a child learning how to tie her shoes, for example, and the survival time would be the age at which she masters this task. Survival data is different from any of the topics we have described so far. At the time of the data analysis, not all of the subjects' data has been completely observed for the event of interest. This is called *censoring*. We describe a number of examples of time-to-event data and different types of censoring in this chapter. Survival curves graphically depict the time-to-event data for a data sample, much as a histogram does in elementary statistics. There are some simple statistical comparisons we can make of survival curves. We describe a regression model in Chapter 12 used to model survival curves with several explanatory variables in a regression setting.

11.1 Censoring

Survival analysis is a collection of statistical methods to model the time it takes for an individual to achieve a specified event. The event could be death, as the name implies, or something less dramatic, such as how long it takes to complete a Master's degree, or how long it takes a legislature to pass a bill into law. We provide a number of other examples in this section.

The study of survival data stands apart from other statistical topics because of *censoring*. Specifically, the exact time of the event for every individual under study may not be available to us at the time of the analysis. There are different types of censoring, as the following examples illustrate.

It is often useful to think of the time line traveling from left to right. The most common type of censoring is called *right censoring*: the left end point, the start of the time line, is known, but the right end point may not have yet occurred at the time we examine the data. The amount of time students spend in a degree program is one example. We know the date when they were admitted. Some students will breeze through and complete all their requirements early. Others will take longer. Some will either drop out or continue working at a slower pace. When it comes time to study the data on time to degree completion, many will already have graduated, but there will also be some who have not yet completed their degrees. We can't tell if and when they ever will. Those who have not yet completed the program at the time of the examination of their data are said to be right censored: we know when they began, but the graduation event may not yet have occurred.

> In right censoring we know the starting time, but the end point may not yet have been reached by all subjects.

The study of HIV involves another type of censoring. Sometimes we can trace a patient's initial infection to a single blood transfusion or sexual contact. In this case we know the start of the infection. Sometimes we do not. For some we may know only that the infection occurred before some date when the infection was first detected. In this case, the left end point of the disease progression time line is said to be *left censored* because we do not know the starting date, only that it occurred before the date of the HIV diagnosis.

Perhaps we can trace the patient's initial HIV infection to one of a series of transfusions or sexual contacts occurring over a period of time. In this case we might say the left end point is *interval censored* because it could have occurred at any point within the time interval.

The time of progression from HIV infection to AIDS often involves another interval censoring. Some AIDS-defining events can only be determined by a blood test, such as when the patient's count of CD4+ cells falls below the threshold value of 200. The CD4+ counts are not monitored continuously, and these values are known only at discrete testing times. If one lab value is above the threshold and the subsequent value is below 200, then we do not know exactly when the threshold was reached. The threshold of 200 could have been passed at any time in between the two adjacent lab dates. In other words, in this examination of the progression from HIV infection to AIDS, both the starting and ending time points may be interval censored.

Here is another example combining different types of censoring. Let us consider the age at which children learn to tie their shoes. A psychologist decides to sit in at a day-care facility for a period of six months to watch the children. During the six-month observation period, some children will learn to tie their shoes, and their exact ages of acquiring the skill will be known. Some children will already know how to tie their shoes when the psychologist arrives, and their ages will be censored on the left. Similarly, some children will still not have this skill when the psychologist's observation period ends and these children will be right censored.

These are examples of the most common types of censoring. An important assumption we make about censoring is the observation of censored or not is unrelated to the actual, unobserved event time.

> We assume whether or not a subject is censored is independent of the actual time to the event.

It is essential to get at the root cause of censoring. In a clinical trial of a new medical treatment, suppose patients were censored because they dropped out and their event times were not recorded. The data would be more difficult to analyze if those patients most likely to drop out were also the ones who were doing very well (or perhaps were very poorly). In either of these cases, we would say the study has *informative censoring*. That is, having a censored observation tells us something about the unobserved outcome.

Instead, in the analysis of survival data, we assume censoring is noninformative and contains no useful information concerning the true event times. Noninformative censoring might occur if the reason for observations being censored had nothing to do with the actual event time. For example, censored patients might have moved to another city or perhaps the statisticians had to meet a deadline and the patients still under study were censored at the time of the data analysis.

We have described most of these different types of censoring, but by far the most common is right censoring with a known (left) starting end point. Right-censored data has received the largest amount of statistical theoretical development and also has the largest amount of software available to analyze the data. Before we talk about software, we need to describe the survival curve.

11.2   The Survival Curve and its Estimate

The *survival curve* estimates the proportion of subjects who have already experienced their event by a given time. Just as we would draw a histogram to examine graphically a new set of data, plotting a survival curve is usually the first step we take when we examine right-censored survival data. A survival curve begins at 1 (or 100%) at time zero and continues to drop in a series of steps. A survival curve can be flat in places, but it can never rise. The estimate of the survival curve is sometimes called the *product limit* or *Kaplan–Meier curve* and is attributed to E. L. Kaplan and Paul Meier who published this method in 1958.

A typical example of a pair of survival curves is given in Fig. 11.1. The data given in Table 11.1 presents the remission times for patients with acute myelogenous leukemia (AML). The outcome is not survival, but the length of time (in weeks) before their symptoms return. Notice we are not measuring time to death of these patients, but rather the time it takes for their leukemia symptoms to return following treatment. The patients received one of two different treatments for their AML: either maintenance of their treatment or no additional treatments.

Initially, at time zero, all patients are in remission. As time progresses, most of these patients relapse. This figure estimates the proportion of patients in remission at each time point. The upper curve is for the treatment-maintained group of patients, so we can conclude these patients will generally have longer remission times. At any time point, we see a greater proportion of treatment-maintained patients remained relapse-free. In Section 11.3 we examine these data again and perform tests of statistical significance comparing the two curves. For the moment, we can see treatment maintenance is better and results in longer remission times. At any remission time,

Table 11.1 Length of remission time, in weeks, for AML patients who were either on maintained treatment or not. Every patient has an indicator of whether their observed time was censored and they were still in remission (0) or whether they had relapsed and the time of their disease recurrence was known (1).

Treatment maintained											
9	1	13	1	13	0	18	1	23	1	28	0
31	1	34	1	45	0	48	1	161	0		
Treatment not maintained											
5	1	5	1	8	1	8	1	12	1	16	0
23	1	27	1	30	1	33	1	43	1	45	1

Available in **R** as `aml` in the `survival` package
Source: Embury *et al.* (1977).

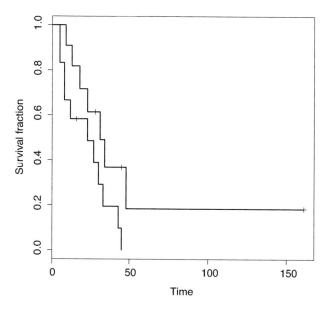

Figure 11.1 Kaplan–Meier survival curves for the AML data in Table 11.1. The upper line is for the treatment-maintained group. The code to draw this figure is given in Output 11.1.

shortly after the start of this study, there are always a greater proportion of treatment maintained patients who have not had progression of their disease.

There are two additional features of the graph worth mentioning in Fig. 11.1. One of these is the small vertical marks. These indicate the locations of the censored observations. This is an optional feature and is not always performed in practice. The inclusion of these small marks allows the reader to see the distribution of censored observations. If there are many censored observations and these occur very early in

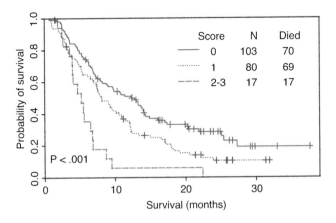

Figure 11.2 Survival of three groups of cancer patients.
Source: Wheler *et al.* (2009).

the study, then this is indicative of inadequate follow-up time. Similarly, if there are many more censored observations in one treatment group, this indicates censoring may not be independent of outcome, a key assumption we stated in the previous section. In the present study, neither of these appears to be a problem.

A second feature of survival curves is the tendency for our eyes to concentrate on the long upper tail extending to the right of this figure. The nonmaintained group has a survival curve dropping to zero, but the maintained group does not. Does this indicate a long-term cure? No, because the long tail to the right only indicates the single longest remission time was censored. That is, the long tail to the right is based on only one observation. If the longest observation is censored, then the survival curve does not go all the way to zero. As you can see, we need to pay more attention to the portion of the survival curve in the upper left corner where most of the data is concentrated. As the curve extends to the right there will be fewer observations.

Figure 11.2 presents a published set of survival curves for three groups of cancer patients enrolled in a Phase I clinical trial. A Phase I trial studies a new drug in its first use in humans. Such studies are experimental in nature, so these trials typically enroll patients who have failed other conventional treatments. Indeed, as we see in Fig. 11.2, few of these patients survived two years.

The authors of this study divided their patients into different groups by assigning a score based on disease severity. We can clearly see those patients who had lower scores survived longer. Most of the censoring occurred in the longest-surviving group. The figure contains details on how many patients were in each of the three groups and how many died. The *p*-value in this figure tests the null hypothesis the patients were sampled from populations with identical survival characteristics. In Section 11.3 we describe how this statistical test was performed.

Consider next a hypothetical situation in which a new therapy is being compared to a conventional treatment with survival times plotted in Fig. 11.3. The new method (such as a heart transplant or experimental cancer treatment) has considerable risk and

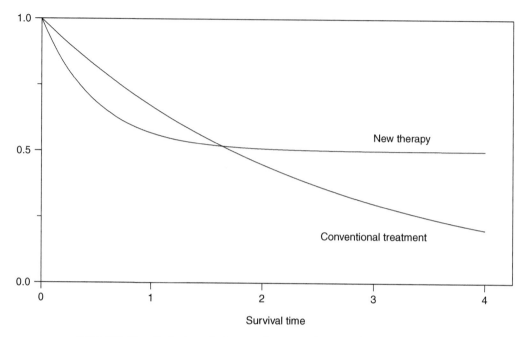

Figure 11.3 Hypothetical survival curves for a new therapy and conventional treatment.

there is a high rate of mortality associated with it. But once patients survive the initial stress, they appear to do much better than those receiving the conventional therapy. Which procedure would you prefer?

This figure presents a difficult situation in which it is not at all clear which is the better group. Compare Fig. 11.2 with Fig. 11.3. Sometimes survival curves may be different, but when they cross as in Fig. 11.3, neither population has a higher survival fraction at all times. A test of statistical significance for comparing survival curves is described in the following section, but this method only tests whether curves are different.

Let us end this section with a description of the Kaplan–Meier method used to construct a survival curve with censored data. Consider the small data set with the following survival times observed for eight subjects

$$1 \quad 2.5+ \quad 3 \quad 3 \quad 3+ \quad 4 \quad 4.5+ \quad 6$$

where a plus + sign indicates a right-censored value.

Table 11.2 shows how to construct a Kaplan–Meier estimate of the survival curve for these data. The number of subjects at risk at any specified time is the number of individuals who are known to have their event times at this time or later. So, at time 1, all eight subjects were considered to be at risk for their events. At time 2.5, there was a censored observation. Censored observations are part of the risk set and denominator, but are not event times, so no computation is done at this time value. At time 3 there were six individuals at risk. It is not known whether the "2.5+" person had their event at time 3 or later, so this subject is not considered to be at risk at time 3.

Table 11.2 Construction of the Kaplan–Meier estimate of the survival curve.

			Event times					
	1	2.5+	3	3	3+	4	4.5+	6
Number at risk	8	—	6		—	3	—	1
Number of events	1	—	2		—	1	—	1
Estimated Pr[event]	1/8	—	1/3		—	1/3	—	1
Estimated Pr[no event]	7/8	—	2/3		—	2/3	—	0
K–M estimate	7/8	—	$7/8 \times 2/3$ $= 7/12$		—	$7/8 \times 2/3 \times 2/3$ $= 7/18$	—	0

Survival fraction

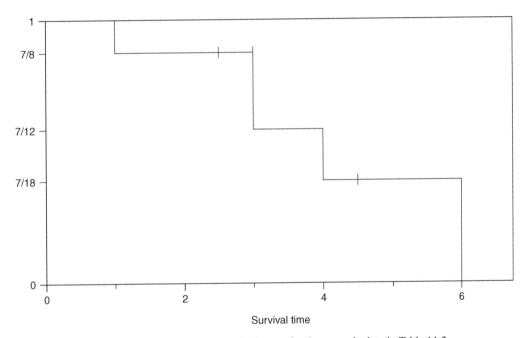

Figure 11.4 The Kaplan–Meier survival curve for the example data in Table 11.2.

The two individuals with events at time 3 are combined. The "Number of events" entry in this table shows these as two events at a single time. All other survival times indicate a single event. Again, censored times are not event times, and these are not considered. The censored 3+ time is considered to have occurred after the two events occurring at time 3.

The estimated probability of an event at each time point is

$$\text{Pr}[\text{event}] = \frac{\text{Number of events}}{\text{Number at risk}}$$

at every event time. This probability is zero where there are no events, such as at a censored time.

Similarly, the probability of no event is

$$\Pr[\,\text{no event}\,] = 1 - \Pr[\,\text{event}\,].$$

Finally, the probability of surviving up to any given time is the product of all the survival probabilities up to this point. This is the product-limit (Kaplan–Meier) estimate of the survival curve. The actual survival curve is plotted in Fig. 11.4.

The key point to remember about plotting survival curves is the curve drops at event times but is flat at censored times and other nonevent times. Whether the longest survival time is censored determines whether the survival curve falls to zero or not. This point was also made in the discussion of Fig. 11.1. We next show how to statistically compare two survival curves.

11.3   The Log-Rank Test

The log-rank test is one of the oldest and most popular methods for comparing two survival curves. The approach is nonparametric. The null hypothesis is that groups of subjects are sampled from the same population. The alternative hypothesis is that the population survival curves are different. The test is suitable for testing data from the example in Fig. 11.3. It does not help us determine which groups is better. It only detects if the groups are different.

Let us illustrate the code comparing the two groups in the AML data given in Output 11.1. The `survival` library has to be installed before using it. The `plot(survfit...)` code produces the pair of survival curves in Fig. 11.1. The `Surv` function creates a *survival object* in **R**. This function has two arguments: the time and the censoring indicator. The function `survdiff` compares the survival times and provides a *p*-value for the null hypothesis the groups are different.

The log-rank test is a comparison of the observed and expected counts in a series of 2×2 tables. Every time an event occurs in either of the two patient groups, we construct a 2×2 table. So, for example, at 23 weeks there was one event in both groups. At this time there were also six patients at risk in the treatment-maintained group and seven patients at risk in the nonmaintained group. We summarize this information in a 2×2 table.

	Treatment maintained	Nonmaintained control
Events	1	1
No events	5	6
Patients at risk	6	7

We can also calculate the expected counts in this table just as we do when we compute the Pearson chi-squared test. Under the null hypothesis, events occur independently of group membership, so the observed counts and expected values should be close.

Output 11.1 Code to produce Fig. 11.1 and compare remission times in the AML data.

```
> library(survival)                # install this library first
> aml <- read.table(file = "AML.txt", header = T)
> aml[1:3,]                        # print a few lines
   time cens group
1    5    1    0
2    5    1    0
3    8    1    0
>
> #                                    Draw Figure 11.1
> plot(survfit(Surv(time, cens) ~ group, data = aml),
+        lwd = 2,  mark.time = TRUE, cex.lab = 1.5,
+        xlab = "Time", ylab = "Survival fraction")

>
> #   Log-rank or Mantel-Haenszel test
> survdiff(Surv(time, cens) ~ group, data = aml)
Call:
survdiff(formula = Surv(time, cens) ~ group, data = aml)

         N Observed Expected (O-E)^2/E (O-E)^2/V
group=0 12      11     7.31      1.86       3.4
group=1 11       7    10.69      1.27       3.4

 Chisq= 3.4  on 1 degrees of freedom, p= 0.0653
>
> #   Peto & Peto modification of the Gehan-Wilcoxon test
> survdiff(Surv(time, cens) ~ group, data = aml, rho = 1)
Call:
survdiff(formula = Surv(time, cens) ~ group, data = aml, rho = 1)

         N Observed Expected (O-E)^2/E (O-E)^2/V
group=0 12    7.18     4.88     1.081      2.78
group=1 11    3.85     6.14     0.859      2.78

 Chisq= 2.8  on 1 degrees of freedom, p= 0.0955
```

There will be one such 2×2 table for every event time in the data. We only need a way to combine these tables. Let o_i be the observed number of events in the upper left corner of each 2×2 table, and let e_i denote the corresponding expected count under the null hypothesis of independence.

The test of survival difference in `survdiff` is based on the statistic

$$\sum_i w_i(o_i - e_i),$$

which adds all of these differences using different nonnegative weights, w_i.

The log-rank or *Mantel–Haenszel test* sets $w_i = 1$ for all values of i. This is the default method in `survdiff`, also obtained setting `rho = 0`. The Peto–Peto test sets w_i equal to the Kaplan–Meier survival fraction estimate at time $t = i$. This test is obtained setting `rho = 1`. In the latter case, more weight is given to differences between the observed and expected counts early, when more data is available.

> The log-rank test compares the difference of observed and
> expected numbers of events at every event time.

Under the null hypothesis of identical population survival curves, events will occur independently in the two groups. More precisely, events are more likely to occur in proportion to the number of subjects at risk in the two groups. This corresponds to subjects in both groups being sampled from the same population survival curve.

Under this null hypothesis, the log-rank statistic should have a value near zero. Values far from zero indicate one group has too many events when few are expected under the model of independence. Similarly, the opposite could also occur, so this is a two-tailed test.

The log-rank statistic also needs to be normalized by its standard deviation. This is done for us in `survdiff` for two choices of weights w_i giving p-values of either 0.0653 or 0.0955, depending on the choice of `rho` we use.

Did you notice how the log-rank and Wilcoxon tests are nonparametric? Nowhere did we need to know the actual times at which the events occurred. In the computation of these statistics we only need to know the number of subjects at risk when an event occurs in either of the two groups. More specifically, we only need the ranked order in which these events happened. Similarly, the p-values for these tests will remain unchanged if we take logs of survival times or otherwise transform these in a way to maintain the order of the events.

A hard question to answer is whether the censored patients dropped out of the study for reasons related to their outcome. Did their health improve and then they quit, or did they leave their treatment because it wasn't working for them? More generally, is there information in the censoring? Sometimes we can't know the answer to these questions. Nevertheless, an important assumption is censoring is independent of the ultimate survival time.

Another difficult question is the resolution of the comparison of survival curves in Fig. 11.3. These curves cross and may be statistically different using the log-rank test. The log-rank test tells us only whether these curves are different; it does not indicate which, if any, is better. We need to make that difficult decision.

In Chapter 12 we describe a regression method for modeling censored survival times to include the effects of covariate information.

11.4   Exercises

11.1   Why can't we compare right-censored survival times using a t-test?

11.2   Suppose we transformed the survival times using log(time) or time squared. Would this affect the comparison of survival data using the log-rank test? Why?

11.3   In Fig. 11.3, which group would you prefer to be in?

11.4.1   Cancer of the Bile Duct

Cancer of the bile duct (Cholangiocarcinoma) is a terrible disease, and most patients die within a year of their diagnosis. A group of patients with this disease were randomized to two treatment groups at the Mayo clinic (see Table 11.3). One group was treated with radiation and 5-fluorouracil (5-FU). This is a common treatment regime for many types of cancers. The second group was left as untreated with a placebo.

What do you see when you compare the two different treatment groups? Is there a difference between the shapes of the survival curves? Can you see a survival advantage to one group or the other? Is there one group you or a loved one would prefer to belong to?

What can you say about a disease if the active treatment is not much better than doing nothing at all? Is the lack of an active treatment ethical for the patients in the control group? Is it ever ethical to assign a placebo to patients? These are hard questions we should consider when performing medical research. We cannot ethically randomize patients to one of several different treatments unless we honestly do not

Table 11.3 Survival times (Surv), in days, of patients treated for bile duct cancer. Censoring is indicated by (Cens = 0); and the death of the patient by (Cens = 1). Patients were treated with either placebo (Trt = 1) or radiation and 5-FU (Trt = 0).

Surv	Cens	Trt	Surv	Cens	Trt	Surv	Cens	Trt	Surv	Cens	Trt
57	1	0	58	1	0	74	1	0	79	1	0
89	1	0	98	1	0	101	1	0	104	1	0
110	1	0	118	1	0	125	1	0	132	1	0
154	1	0	159	1	0	188	1	0	203	1	0
257	1	0	257	1	0	431	1	0	461	1	0
497	1	0	723	1	0	747	1	0	1313	1	0
2636	1	0									
30	1	1	67	1	1	79	0	1	82	0	1
95	0	1	148	1	1	170	1	1	171	1	1
176	1	1	193	1	1	200	1	1	221	1	1
243	1	1	261	1	1	262	1	1	263	1	1
399	1	1	414	1	1	446	1	1	446	0	1
464	1	1	777	1	1						

Source: Fleming *et al.* (1980).

Table 11.4 Survival of centenarians.

Age at last birthday	Number at risk	Deaths	Number censored
100	52,947	20,845	2,256
101	29,846	12,213	1,317
102	16,316	6,799	716
103	8,801	3,852	392
104	4,557	2,030	193
105	2,334	1,169	103
106	1,062	500	63
107	499	271	9
108	219	129	16
109	74	46	1
110	27	24	
111	3	2	
112	1	1	

Sources: Kannisto (1988) and Zelterman (1992).

know whether one is better than the others. This principle of equally valid treatments is called *equipoise*.

11.4.2   Survival of Centenarians

What are the limits of human longevity? Are there any limits? These are important questions to demographers, who debate the existence of such limits and what they might be. Part of the answer may lie in a study of survival of very old people. An example of such data appears in Table 11.4.

A *centenarian* is a person who is 100 years old. The data represents the survival of female centenarians from 13 countries in northern Europe and Scandinavia. This data was carefully collected by Kannisto (1988), who was concerned about individuals intentionally overstating their age in order to claim to be centenarians.

Construct a survival curve for these data. Is this the right way to display this data? The ages begin at 100, so it is best to use this as the starting value for the time axis. The survival curve falls very quickly. Why is that? Perhaps the vertical survival axis should plot the log of the survival proportion. If we do that, the survival curve is always negative. Why is that?

Construct the survival curve following the example of Table 11.2. Plot values of Pr[event] in this table against age at last birthday. Do these probabilities generally increase or decrease over time? Why do you think this may be the case? These probabilities estimate the *hazard function*, important in models described in the following chapter.

Does there appear to be a limit of longevity? Can it be estimated from these data? Can this be done without extrapolating from the observed data?

12 Proportional Hazards Regression

Much of the language of survival analysis dates back to the 1600s with the early Dutch traders. Ships would leave Europe on a long and dangerous journey to India and China. When they returned with spices and silk they brought great wealth and fortune to sailors who risked their lives and the bankers who invested in the ship and its crew. Along the way they might have to contend with storms, pirates, and illness. Sometimes traders failed to return and were never heard from again, leaving behind widows, orphans, and financial ruin for their backers. Survival was always part of the discussion in planning such ventures. The need to spread the risks involved in these journeys gave rise to the insurance industry.

Survival analysis uses a lot of the language of life insurance. If we think of life insurance as a bet, then we also need to think of the company taking the other side of this bet. *Actuaries* are statisticians who assess the risks and then set the rates commensurately for the insurance company. If an actuary overestimates the risk, then the company will charge high rates and may lose customers. If the actuary underestimates the risks, the company faces financial disaster should claims exceed their ability to pay. Many of the terms used in this chapter will be familiar to actuaries and were originally developed by them. The hazard function is a natural way to describe risk. It leads us to a popular and effective regression method for modeling survival data.

12.1 The Hazard Function

The *hazard function* (also called the *failure rate*) is a conditional probability. The hazard is the probability of having an event occur at the next instant of time for a subject who has not yet had the event occur. The company selling life insurance wants to know the probability those insured will die within the next year given they are alive at the beginning of the year. In our use, we define the hazard to be the probability of the event occurring during the next small instant of time for any individual, provided it has not yet happened.

> The hazard at a given time is the probability an event will occur
> in the next instant for a person who has not already experienced the event.

Intuitively, large values of the hazard mean the event is likely to occur soon. Larger values of the hazard function also mean the survival curve is falling faster. Similarly, if the survival curve is falling slowly, then the hazard is low.

The mathematical definition of the hazard function at time t is

$$\text{hazard}(t) = \Delta^{-1} \frac{\Pr[\text{ event happens between } t \text{ and } t + \Delta \,]}{\Pr[\text{ event has not happened by time } t \,]}$$

for values of Δ close to zero.

This expression should look like a derivative in calculus. The hazard is closely related to the rate of decrease of the survival curve. If the survival curve is falling quickly then the hazard function is larger.

We won't be needing this formula, but here is some intuition about what it measures. The probability in the denominator restricts our attention to only those individuals who have not experienced the event by time t. This is the proportion of people at risk, also described in Table 11.2.

The hazard function is not the probability we will live to be a certain age. Instead, the actuarial hazard is the probability we will not live one more year. The actuary's hazard can tell us the probability of a 100-year-old person dying within the next year. The hazard does not easily tell us the probability of our living to be 100, however. An annual estimate for the hazard function of centenarians is constructed in Section 11.4.2. The hazard used in this chapter is the probability a subject will experience the event within the next instant of time. For actuaries, the instant Δ is one year; for us, the instant is very small.

Before we go on, it would be useful to look at the actuarial hazard function for our whole lifespan. A great deal of the life insurance industry is based on the human hazard, so this has been studied for many years and measured with great care. There are also separate estimates of the hazard rates for men and women, different racial groups, and smokers and nonsmokers. In Fig. 12.1 we plot the hazard function for the all-combined US population, up to 80 years. The US Centers for Disease Control offers a variety of resources to learn more about these data.

Figure 12.1 is not entirely useful to us except to emphasize the interpretation of the hazard. The relatively larger hazard at the lowest ages illustrates infant mortality. It is not surprising the hazard rises at older ages as the population increasingly experiences the risks of heart disease, cancer, kidney failure, and other diseases associated with aging. Most persons seeing this figure are surprised to learn the lowest value occurs between ages 10 and 11. This minimum of the hazard corresponds to the age at which humans have the greatest force of vitality (as opposed to mortality) and have the greatest probability of living one more year. Sadly, most of us will view this figure and probably realize our prime years have long passed.

The hazard function in this chapter does not use the data in this figure. For the statistical analysis of survival data, we are concerned with selected populations, viewed not over their entire lifetimes, but rather, over a relatively short period of time.

In a single population, we can estimate the hazard function by the $\Pr[\text{ event }]$ in Table 11.2. This is not very useful, because we frequently have several populations

Hazard × 1000

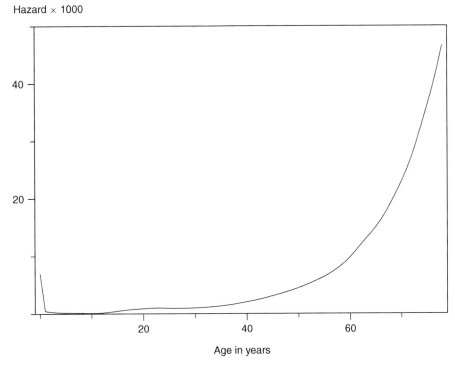

Figure 12.1 Human lifetime hazard function for the combined 2003 US population.

we want to compare and, as we see in Section 12.2, we want to include covariate effects from additional information collected on each subject.

12.2   The Model of Proportional Hazards Regression

Having a large value of our hazard function is a bad thing, unless perhaps we are talking about the hazard function for time to winning the lottery. Otherwise, a large hazard function means there is a greater risk of the event occurring in the next time interval. Larger hazards are associated with even greater imminent risk.

The model of proportional hazards uses this idea. We begin with a *baseline hazard* modeling the same underlying risk associated with all subjects in the data. Much as the intercept is common to all observations in a linear regression, the baseline hazard function $h(t)$ is roughly a measure of the average hazard for all subjects at time t.

The variations in individual hazards are expressed as multiples of the baseline $h(t)$. Specifically, the model of *proportional hazards* specifies the hazard $h_i(t)$ for the ith subject is expressible as

$$h_i(t) = C_i\, h(t), \tag{12.1}$$

where each C_i is a positive number depending on the risk factors of the ith subject.

In (12.1), the C_i depend on information collected on the ith individual. The C_i do not depend on time t. The baseline hazard $h(t)$ is the same for everybody and does not depend on characteristics measured on individuals. Similarly, we usually do not concern ourselves with the baseline hazard $h(t)$ because it is the same for everyone.

In other words, at each time t, every subject's hazard function is proportional to every other's according to (12.1). The proportion C_i is a function of the unique explanatory values measured on the ith individual.

> The model of proportional hazards assumes each individual's hazard is a constant multiple of the hazard rate common to all.

When we model survival data using proportional hazards, we examine the values of the positive multipliers C_i. Values of C_i greater than 1 indicate a greater risk of the event than described by the baseline hazard and a generally shorter time to the event. Values of C_i between 0 and 1 indicate a lowered risk and longer time to event. We next describe a regression modeling the value of each individual's C_i.

Proportional hazards regression, sometimes called *Cox regression*,[1] is a way of modeling the multiplier C_i of the hazard function in terms of covariates. The covariates or risk factors are combined in a linear fashion much in the way we have been modeling linear, logistic, or Poisson regression.

Proportional hazards regression is performed in **R** using coxph. This routine has similar syntax to lm and glm. It is described in the following section.

In the proportional hazards model, the baseline hazard $h(t)$ acts as an intercept and is the same for every subject. Consequently, we do not usually talk about the baseline hazard. Instead, proportional hazards regression only looks at models of the positive multiplier C_i. Specifically, in proportional hazards regression, we seek to assess the effects of covariate values $x_1, \ldots, x_k$ measured on all subjects and see how these change the multiplier C_i.

Because C_i must be a positive number, we usually assume a log-link and set

$$\log C_i = \beta_1 x_1 + \cdots + \beta_k x_k \tag{12.2}$$

for regression coefficients $\beta_1, \ldots, \beta_k$ estimated by coxph in **R**.

As an example of the interpretation of this model, if β_1 is positive, then increasing the value of x_1 means an increase in the hazard and a correspondingly shorter survival time or time to event. This is somewhat against our intuition. An increase in the hazard means the survival is falling faster and survival is shorter. Remember we are modeling the hazard of survival times and not the survival times themselves. Larger hazards mean shorter survival times.

There is no intercept in the proportional hazards regression model given in (12.2). An intercept in this model would be the same for all observations and would then be absorbed into the baseline hazard function $h(t)$.

---

[1] David R. Cox, a British statistician, published this idea in 1972.

Let us describe the example of proportional hazards regression in the AML data from Table 11.1. The model for proportional hazards in this data is

$$h_i(t) = e^{g\beta} h(t)$$

where the group indicator $g = 0$ or 1 signifying membership and $h(t)$ is the baseline hazard function shared by all individuals.

Specifically, we can write this model as

$$h_i(t) = \begin{cases} h(t) & \text{for treatment discontinued (group } g = 0) \\ e^{\beta} h(t) & \text{for treatment continued (group } g = 1), \end{cases}$$

where the regression coefficient β is estimated in the following section. The baseline hazard function $h(t)$ is common to all patients, and we generally do not concern ourselves with this.

If $\beta > 0$, then treatment continuation results in a higher hazard, and this will result in shorter times to relapse. Similarly, if $\beta < 0$, then continuation of treatment is beneficial. As with other regression models, the null hypothesis is $\beta = 0$ corresponding to no difference in treatment schedule.

We next fit a proportional hazards regression models in **R**.

12.3   Proportional Hazards Regression in R

Let us begin by fitting the model of proportional hazards to the the AML data from Table 11.1. The code and results appear in Output 12.1. The syntax of coxph is similar

---

Output 12.1 Proportional hazards regression for the AML data.

```
> library(survival)               # install this library first
> aml <- read.table(file = "AML.txt", header = T)
> aml[1:3,]                        # print a few lines
  time cens group
1   5    1    0
2   5    1    0
3   8    1    0
> coxph(Surv(time, cens) ~ group, data = aml)
Call:
coxph(formula = Surv(time, cens) ~ group, data = aml)

        coef exp(coef) se(coef)     z     p
group -0.916     0.400    0.512 -1.79 0.074

Likelihood ratio test=3.38  on 1 df, p=0.0658
n= 23, number of events= 18
```

---

to `survdiff` seen in Output 11.1. As with `survdiff`, we need to create a survival object in **R** using the `Surv` function. The survival object requires we specify the name of the time variable and the censoring variable. The linear model in coxph is written in a familiar manner.

The estimated regression coefficient for `group` is -0.916 indicating the subjects with group $= 1$ (treatment maintained) had a lower hazard and corresponding longer remission times. The statistical significance for this regression coefficient is 0.074 giving evidence that the differences in estimated hazard rates are unlikely to have happened by chance alone. Remember there is no intercept in proportional hazards regression.

The `Likelihood ratio test` has $p = 0.0658$ providing a similar degree of statistical significance. Both p-values are comparable to the two values obtained from the log-rank test in Output 11.1. The method of proportional hazards regression agrees with those two previous examinations of this data and provides about the same amount of moderate evidence continued treatment is beneficial for prolonging remission times in AML.

The *hazard ratio* is calculated as

$$\exp(-0.916) = 0.4001,$$

showing treatment-maintained individuals with group $= 1$ values have a hazard 0.400 times as large as those with group $= 0$. This is the estimated value of C_i in (12.1). The lowered hazard for group $i = 1$ patients is associated with longer times to relapse. We also have $C_0 = 1$ (group $= 0$) corresponding to the baseline hazard ratio.

An important diagnostic for proportional hazards is to employ plotted survival curves to see if different groups do not cross. We see this is indeed the case for this data in Fig. 11.1. If one group has a consistently higher hazard rate, then its survival curve will always be lower. Similarly, proportional hazards regression may not detect a difference in the crossing survival curves in Fig. 11.3 and such a figure is an indication of invalid assumptions of the method.

Output 12.2 Code to plot martingale and deviance residuals in Fig. 12.2.

```
ph.out <- coxph(Surv(time, cens) ~ group, data = aml)

#  Martingale residuals
plot(jitter(aml$group), ph.out$residuals, xlab = "Jittered group",
     main = "Martingale residuals",
     ylab = "", pch = 19, cex = 1.5, cex.lab = 1.25)

#  Deviance residuals
plot(jitter(aml$group), resid(ph.out, type = "deviance"),
     xlab = "Jittered group", ylab = "",
     main = "Deviance residuals",
     pch = 19, cex = 1.5, cex.lab = 1.25)
```

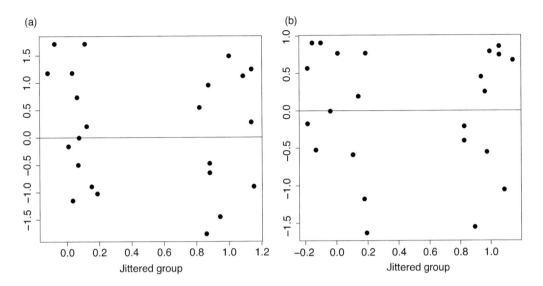

Figure 12.2 (a) Deviance residuals and (b) martingale residuals in proportional hazards regression.

In addition to the estimated regression coefficients, there are two types of residuals in proportional hazards regression. These are the martingale and deviance residuals. Output 12.2 contains the code to obtain these and they are plotted in Fig. 12.2 against the jittered group. Jittering adds a small amount of random noise to the group variable in order to see if there is any pattern. Jittering was introduced in Section 2.5.2.

The residuals have different definitions but should not differ greatly in value. They behave approximately as standard normal if the model fits well, and values larger than 2 in absolute value might be suspect. Figure 12.2 does not reveal any outliers or unusual observations using either definition of residual.

12.4 Exercises

12.1 Why can't we use a linear regression to compare right-censored survival times with covariates?

12.2 Are the hazards proportional if the survival curves cross, as in Fig. 11.3?

12.4.1 Survival of Halibut

A halibut is a large and tasty fish sought by sportsmen. Halibut travel in huge schools. The schools are so large these can be tracked in satellite images. This technology can be exploited by commercial fishermen who can quickly harvest great numbers on hooked lines which can be miles long. Consequently, halibut fishing must be carefully regulated to prevent the eventual depletion of their stocks. To inform this regulation, halibut populations have been studied in detail. One suggestion is to impose the size limit of 32 inches. This regulation only works if the smaller fish are still alive when returned to the sea, motivating the collection of the data in this section.

Halibut have an ear bone with rings allowing us to accurately estimate their age just as we would with trees. When young, halibut have one eye on either side of their heads and swim up-and-down or perpendicular to the surface of the water. At about six months of age, halibut will begin to swim flat with the light-colored side toward the bottom and a much darker side on top. At the time they make this transition, the eye on the bottom side of the head moves over to the top. The light coloration is for protection from predators looking up toward the surface, and the two eyes on top help to spot smaller prey above.

What are the determinants of halibut survival once caught? Longer survival translates into fresher fish for the consumer as well as survival of the smaller fish, subsequently returned to the sea. The data set contains 294 lines, one for the survival time of each halibut. Only the first few lines are given in Table 12.1.

For each fish we can learn the following.

- Survival time, measured in hours.
- Censoring indicator: 1 = observed survival time; 0 = censored observation.
- Time the trawl net was towed along the bottom.
- Difference between maximum and minimum depth observed during tow (measured in meters).
- Fork length of halibut (measured in centimeters).
- Handling time (in minutes) between net coming on board vessel and fish placed in holding tanks.
- Logarithm (base e) of total catch of fish in tow.

Table 12.1 The first ten lines of the halibut survival data.

1	209.0	1	30	13	41	8	6.992
2	209.0	1	30	13	44	8	6.992
3	209.0	1	30	13	47	10	6.992
4	209.0	1	30	13	34	10	6.992
5	38.0	1	30	13	40	11	6.992
6	209.0	1	30	13	42	11	6.992
7	140.9	1	30	13	41	12	6.992
8	140.9	1	30	13	30	12	6.992
9	140.1	1	30	1	45	4	4.299
10	208.0	1	30	1	47	5	4.299
⋮			⋮			⋮	

The data originally appeared in Smith *et al.* Ch. 7 of Lange *et al.* (1984), and can be downloaded from Rose *et al.* (2019): https://cdnsciencepub .com/doi/abs/10.1139/cjfas-2018-0350.

Is there evidence that data from a few catches may be pooled together? Similarly, are the survival times listed for individual halibut or is there a single value for a group of fish?

12.4.2 Stanford Heart Transplant Survival

In the early days of heart transplantation, there was an epidemiology study to examine the risks and to see if the procedure was all worthwhile. Subjects were enrolled and randomized to receive a transplant or not. Some subjects who were randomized to receive a transplant died before a donor organ was available. Today we have sophisticated anti-rejection drugs preventing recipients' immune systems from attacking the donor organ. At the time of this study, the mismatch score was important in identifying a close match between donor and recipient. One version of this data is available online as heart in the **R** package survival along with more details and the history of this data set.

Is there evidence the effect of age is not monotone? We would expect the oldest patients would be frail and might not survive the major transplant surgery. The very youngest patients are also vulnerable. A child who needs a heart transplant should be considered to have a different disease than a 60-year-old. Is there evidence the regression on age is not linear? That is, the hazard in age might be "U" shaped with poor survival among those in the extreme lowest and highest ages. Do your martingale residuals indicate any outliers? What makes these individuals stand out?

12.4.3 Primary Biliary Cirrhosis

Primary biliary cirrhosis (PBC) is a disease of the liver characterized by slow loss of bile ducts (bile canaliculi). This results in a buildup of bile, resulting in scarring, fibrosis, cirrhosis, and ultimately liver failure. The disease affects about 1 in 4000 people, mostly women. The current, best treatment is a liver transplant resulting in a 70% 10-year survival.

A randomized clinical trial was conducted between 1974 and 1984 at the Mayo Clinic to see if the use of the drug D-penicillamine would be useful in extending life. In addition, a large proportion of patients developed liver toxicity due to the drugs used to treat their disease. As a result, there are two types of time-to-event end points we can examine in this data: time to toxicity or time to death. Both of these can be modeled as survival times.

In the clinical trial, there were 312 patients randomized to the drug; these patients also have the most complete data. An additional 112 cases were not enrolled in the trial. Some data was collected on them, but much of their data is missing and we should initially concentrate on the 312 who were enrolled in the study.

The data is available as pbc in the **R** package survival. Type help(pbc) for a more detailed explanation of the study and published references to the clinical trial. A complete list of the variables is given in Table 12.2.

Table 12.2 List of variables in the PBC study.

```
case number
survival in days
status: 0=censored, 1=censored due to liver toxicity, 2=death
drug: 1=D-penicillamine, 2=placebo
age in days
sex:  0=male, 1=female
presence of asictes: 0=no 1=yes
presence of hepatomegaly: 0=no 1=yes
presence of spiders  0=no 1=yes
edema: 0=no edema; .5=edema present resolved; 1=edema despite therapy
serum bilirubin in mg/dl
serum cholesterol in mg/dl
albumin in gm/dl
urine copper in ug/day
alkaline phosphatase in U/liter
SGOT in U/ml
triglicerides in mg/dl
platelets per cubic ml / 1000
prothrombin time in seconds
histologic stage of disease
```

Some variables (prothrombin and phosphatase, specifically) are highly significant as explanatory variables of survival. Can you tell whether these are these more indicative of disease progression than of treatment-related outcomes? Specifically, are the values of these variables different in the treated and placebo groups?

Is the rate of censoring different in the two different groups? Was there more censoring due to liver toxicity in the treated group than in the placebo patients? You might use logistic regression to see if censoring due to toxicity was related to any of the other explanatory variables. Was the drug effective in prolonging survival?

12.4.4   Multiple Myeloma

Myeloma is a disease of the immune system in the bone marrow. Presently, it is incurable but symptom-free survival can be achieved with a variety of treatments. Patients can be expected to live four to five years.

The data is from a report on survival data from a study of 65 patients treated with alkylating agents. Of these patients, 48 died during the study and 17 were still alive at the time of the data analysis. The variables given in this data set are listed in Table 12.3.

Blood urea nitrogen (BUN) is a measure of kidney function. Urea is produced by the liver and cleared from the blood by the kidneys. Hemoglobin (HGB) is an important component of blood involved in transporting gases to be exchanged in the lungs.

Table 12.3 List of variables in the multiple myeloma data set.

```
Survival time, measured in months
Censoring indicator (0=alive, 1=dead)
BUN at time of diagnosis, log scale
Hemoglobin at time of diagnosis
Normal platelets at diagnosis (1=normal, 0=abnormal)
Age, in years, at time of diagnosis
WBC at time of diagnosis, log scale
Fractures at time of diagnosis (0=none, 1=present)
Percent of plasma cells in the bone marrow, PBM, on log scale
Proteinuria: Protein in the urine
Serum calcium at time of diagnosis
```

Available as myeloid in the **R** package survival.

Examine the data using proportional hazards models. Notice BUN is highly significant in explaining survival times. HGB is a little less useful in this role. Are these variables correlated with other explanatory variables? Can you tell whether survival is a general overall decline in health or a function of only these two measures?

There is one extreme outlier found using martingale residuals, but this patient is not at all extreme on the deviance residual scale. Identify this patient and see if you can tell why this observation is unusual.

13 Review of Methods

In the study of statistics we learn a great many different methods, and it is often not readily apparent which is applicable in a given setting. Often the problem with data analysis can be traced back to the choice of which method is most appropriate for the data. This chapter provides a review of the methods from the standpoint of the data analyst.

13.1   The Appropriate Method

A number of different situations are presented here, and the reader is encouraged to think about the appropriate statistical method for each. In each of the following questions, briefly explain the best statistical technique to resolve the question. Specify the null hypothesis in each situation.

13.1 I want to estimate how long it takes for seniors to get back to normal living activities following hip surgery. Does it matter whether the surgery is elective or if it follows an accidental fall and fracture? Some people are climbing ladders within four weeks, but others remain in a wheelchair for the rest of their lives. I also want to investigate the effects of other information including age, sex, Medicaid status, and the need for a home health aide. (What methods should we use? What is the null hypothesis?)

13.2 One of the students tells the following story: Last summer I had a job in a doughnut factory. Those machines would produce a ton of doughnuts every day! My job was to run the machine punching out the holes in the donuts. This worked OK, mostly, but I had to be on the lookout for those few doughnuts with square holes. The number of these were recorded on a daily basis. I was supposed to throw these out, but I secretly took them home and fed them to my dog. By the end of the summer, my dog got sick from eating too many doughnuts. I wondered if there was an increase in the number of square-holed doughnuts as the weather got warmer. Maybe it was worse if the doughnuts were sugar coated. Glazed doughnuts were the worst! Definitely. (Method? Null hypothesis?)

13.3 A political scientist studied how long it took for bills to be passed into law by the state and federal legislatures. Different kinds of bills are introduced into debate:

funding for roads and schools, changes in taxes, and changes in criminal law, as examples. Some bills were quickly passed into law, whereas debate on others continued for years. The political scientist wanted to write an article about the approval process while many bills were still pending. Does the length of the approval process depend on what kind of bill is introduced? Does it matter which political party introduces the bill? (What method is appropriate? What is the null hypothesis?)

13.4   Nobody really cares about the color of car tires. One tire manufacturer suspects darker tires have less grip and take longer to stop on wet pavement. Given data on the shade (measured on a continuous scale) and stopping distance for several brands of tires, how can we test this hypothesis? We tried different tires on different makes and models of cars. (Method? Null hypothesis?)

13.5   Suppose everyone who took a statistics course received a grade of either A or B, without exception. How would we see if grades differed by students' age, sex, major, or number of other courses taken concurrently?

13.6   Most course evaluations are fairly accurate, but there are always a few subjective responses unrelated to the instruction. One professor sometimes gets great evaluations because she wears cool sneakers to class. Another professor sometimes gets poor evaluations because he has a foreign accent. Some professors are simply old and cranky. How can we test whether evaluations differ by required or elective courses?

13.7   The number of housing starts is an important economic indicator. People who buy a new house will also spend a lot of money to furnish it. In many parts of the country, most housing construction begins in the spring. If we had data on the (unadjusted) number of housing starts for each month over many years, how would we create a seasonally adjusted number for each month? Specify the indicator variables you would create and how you would use these in a model.

13.8   We want to compare the response rates following the use of two different antibiotics: One is a standard drug, the other is a new competitor. Each patient's response is classified as improved or not. We know almost all patients will improve even if they are untreated, so a very large clinical trial is needed. As the biostatistician assigned to this project, how are you going to analyze the data? Specifically, what method are you going to use, and what is the null hypothesis?

13.9   In order to study proper diagnostics and drug prescribing practices, we have data on patients including selected information (compliant with HIPPA, the Health Insurance Portability Accountability Act) from their health records. Every prescription is classified as being either proper or improper. We want to see if these (proper/improper) rates are different for male versus female patients, for example, and we want to measure the effects of patient's age, comorbidity, type of health insurance, as well as a lot of other possible covariates. What statistical method do you suggest we use? How would you define your study population?

13.10   Leukemia patients were treated following one of two different medical proto-
cols. They are all disease-free now, but we want to know if their treatment influences
the time until their disease recurs. Some patients remain disease-free for the rest of
their lives. We also want to take into account the effects of any prior treatments,
different ages of the patients, types of health insurance if any, and any comorbidity
conditions. (Method? Hypotheses?)

13.11   Hardly anybody contracts rabies these days, yet in this state there are a couple
of cases every year. How can we test for a trend in the number of cases over the past
five years? (Method? Hypotheses?)

13.12   We want to know if older people are more likely to be cat owners. (Everybody
is either a cat owner or not. You know which you are!) We decided old means anybody
over 25 years old. (Method? Hypotheses?)

13.13   We are in the same situation as in Question 13.12, but we want to use age as a
continuous variable (Method? Hypothesis?)

13.14   In a case-control study, we first identify a number of individuals with a rare
disease and then find a group of otherwise healthy people (controls) with similar
demographic characteristics such as age, race, and sex.
    What statistical method should we use to compare any history of tobacco use
among the cases and controls? What are the null and alternative hypotheses for this
problem?
    Suppose, in the same data, we wanted to compare the level of educational attain-
ment (measured in years) among the cases and controls. What methods should be
used? What are the null and alternative hypotheses?

13.15   In a laboratory study, groups of mice were exposed to different doses of a sus-
pected toxin. Write out the linear logistic regression model expressing the probability
of dying (P) in terms of the dose of exposure.
a.   In terms of what you wrote, what is the null hypothesis, and what is the
     alternative?
b.   Suppose the estimated intercept is -3 and the estimated regression slope on
     Dose is 0.5. Estimate the LD_{50} or Dose lethal to 50% of the mice.

13.2   Other Review Questions

13.16   What is the standard deviation? What does it measure? What is the standard
error? What does it measure? How do these two measures relate to each other?

13.17   What is meant by the use of the "log-link" in Poisson regression? Why is this
needed?

13.18   In the lottery winner data from Section 10.1, suppose we fit a model using the
following code:

```
glm(winners ~ pop, family = poisson, data=lottery)
```

where `winners` is the number of winners and `pop` is the town population in thousands.

Give a mathematical expression for the Poisson mean being fitted. Is this what you wanted to fit? Does this model express the number of winners as proportional to the town's population?

13.19 Part of the output from the program on the previous question includes the following.

```
Coefficients:
            Estimate Std. Error z value Pr(>|z|)
(Intercept) 1.217255   0.182058   6.686 2.29e-11 ***
pop         0.025344   0.005423   4.674 2.96e-06 ***
```

What is the null hypothesis being tested by the `z value` statistic with a value of 4.674? Is this test useful in the present context? Why or why not?

Taken by itself, is the intercept useful in the present example? Briefly explain why or why not.

13.20 In logistic regression, what is meant by the *logit*? Why is it needed? How does this differ from the *probit*? Is there anything you can do using one model but is unavailable to you under the other?

13.21 In the beetle data of Table 8.1, bugs were put in each of six different jars and exposed to different doses of an insecticide. We fit a logistic regression model using the following code.

```
resp <- cbind(died, lived)  # create response values
glm(resp ~ bugs$dose, family = binomial)
```

Write down the mathematical model being fitted with this program.

13.22 Part of the output from the code in Question 13.21 contains the following.

```
Coefficients:
            Estimate Std. Error z value Pr(>|z|)
(Intercept)   -4.898      1.645  -2.977  0.00291 **
bugs$dose      3.964      1.335   2.970  0.00298 **
```

What null hypothesis is being tested by the `z value` statistic with a value of 2.970? Is this address a relevant question?

13.23 Following the output of Question 13.21 , we plot the hat diagonals in Fig. 13.1. Explain what this plot measures and why it is "U" shaped.

13.24 Lymphoma patients will usually respond quickly to chemotherapy, but things can go wrong. Sometimes their response takes a long time, and we may not see it by the time we examine the data. Sometimes the patients don't respond at all, and

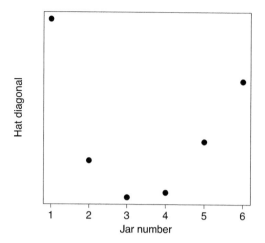

Figure 13.1 Hat diagnostic for logistic regression on insect data.

sometimes they die before responding. Summarize the different kinds of censoring in this setting when we study the time to response.

13.25   Here are some response times, in weeks, where a "+" indicates a censored time. Draw a Kaplan–Meier survival curve for this data and provide as much detail as possible.

3	3+	4	6	10+	12+

13.26   In Question 13.25, a researcher collected much more data than is presented here. Suppose there were 100 additional observations with times shorter than three weeks, and all of these observations were censored. How would the addition of this new data change the estimated survival curve?

   Does the survival curve in the previous question end at zero? Why not?

13.27   In a study of childhood development, we collected data on six-year-old girls and boys along with their weights. By the end of the data collection process, we noticed there were a small number of missing values. There were a lot of children with complete data, but several children were missing either their sex or their weight values.

   What is the best way to estimate a missing weight for a girl or a boy?

   What statistical method can we use to estimate the missing sex of a child from their weight?

13.28   In a large clinical trial of cancer, we noticed some patients responded to the drug and some did not. We want to see if we could characterize these two different types of patients, so we collected data on 500 genetic markers in the laboratory on every subject. We then constructed a total of 500 2×2 tables classifying the numbers of patients who responded (or didn't) and whether or not each of the 500 genes was expressed differently. Every marker was examined in its own 2×2 table. On every 2×2 table we calculated a chi-squared statistic. Of these 500 statistics, 23 of these were found to be statistically significant at the 0.05 level and 6 were statistically significant at the 0.01 level. How do we interpret this finding?

13.29 Here are observations from two groups of observations we want to compare.

Group I: 8   12   97   103
Group II: 19   21   25   27   29   30

Do you prefer a nonparametric test to the t-test for this data? Why? Perform as much of the Wilcoxon rank sum test as you can without a calculator or computer.

With this same data, perform as much of the median test as you can. Set it up, but don't perform any calculations.

13.30 All cases of cancer in Connecticut are recorded and reported to federal agencies as part of the national cancer registry SEER program. We examined these lung cancer rates over the past five years and found New Haven is always worse than the state as a whole. Somebody asked about the *p*-value. What is the most appropriate thing to say?

13.31 Pacemaker batteries are replaced when they fail, or else every two years, whichever comes first. A manufacturer of a new battery makes claims of a lower failure rate. To test this claim, we enrolled a large number of patients into a randomized, double-blind study. When the patients' batteries were replaced, either the old or new battery types were used. At the time of our examination of the data, some batteries will have failed, some will have been replaced after their two-year limit, and some may still be functioning normally in patients.
a. Explain how you will treat each of these three different types of data.
b. Describe a robust statistical method for comparing failure rates of the two types of batteries.
c. How can we account for differences in battery failure rates by patient age, sex, body-mass index, and the age of the pacemaker?

13.32 My friend went to El Salvador and recorded the height and sex of all the third graders in his host village. He came back and performed a linear regression of sex and height, but obtained the unusual residual plot given in Fig. 13.2. He printed and insists there is no problem in his data. Can you help him?

13.33 Last summer we went out into the woods and collected a huge number of ticks. For each, we recorded the environments in which they were found. The environmental data includes such information as wet or dry areas, sunny or shady, rain or fair weather, and in deep grass or under trees. We spent different amounts of time and effort in each of these settings. Only a small number of these ticks tested positive for Lyme disease. We want to present an advisory to hikers about the environments they are likely to find ticks. Describe a statistical analysis to estimate where the infected ticks are likely to occur. Discuss the relative merits of Poisson and logistic regression methodology in this problem.

13.34 We examined families and counted the number of children (under the age of six years) in the household reporting flu symptoms over the past year. We also

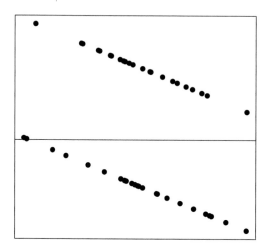

Figure 13.2 What is the problem with these residuals?

recorded the number of adults in the home who smoked, the levels of humidity in the home, and the age of the home. Can we treat each family as an independent binomial sample with $N =$ the number of children and the response variable is the count of symptomatic children?

13.35   I am comparing two survival curves. One goes all the way down to zero at the end, and the second curve stops before reaching zero. How do you explain this?

13.36   For each of 12 Asian countries, I performed a linear regression, modeling per-capita health expenditures (Y) in terms of national population (X). China is much larger than all other nations, so I expect something unusual is going to happen. In fact, the slope is negative when I include all of the data, but the slope becomes positive when I fit the model with all countries except China. What is going on here? Draw a picture to illustrate your explanation.

13.37   I got my Master's thesis data from a brother-in-law of my sister's roommate in Iowa. "He is such a scatter-brained type he probably put some decimal places where they don't belong," she said. I suspect there are some digits reversed, too. I really need to graduate on time, and this is probably the best data available. Is there anything I can do with this? Can you help me? What statistical methods should I be using with this type of data?

Appendix   Statistical Distributions

A.1   Normal Distribution

The **R** function pnorm(x) provides the area to the left of x under the standard normal distribution for $x > 0$. This area is illustrated in Fig. A.1. Examples of the use of this function are given in Section 2.3.

In **R** we obtain these values using pnorm(). Here is an example of its use.

```
> (x <- -3: 3)
[1] -3 -2 -1  0  1  2  3
> pnorm(x)
[1] 0.001349898 0.022750132 0.158655254 0.500000000 0.841344746 0.977249868
[7] 0.998650102
```

There are times when we know the area and need the value of the corresponding normal variate. This is called the *quantile function*. In **R**, the normal quantile is found using qnorm. Here is an example of its use, including the familiar 1.96 value corresponding to a two-tailed critical value for a test with significance level 0.05.

```
> (area <- (1 : 7) / 100)
[1] 0.01 0.02 0.03 0.04 0.05 0.06 0.07
> qnorm(area)
[1] -2.326348 -2.053749 -1.880794 -1.750686 -1.644854 -1.554774 -1.475791
> qnorm(c(0.025, 0.975))    # familiar values
[1] -1.959964  1.959964
```

There are also ways to generate random values from a standard normal distribution using the rnorm function.

```
> rnorm(4)
[1] -1.2389288  0.1887419  0.8208911  0.1838922
```

We obtain different values every time we use rnorm.

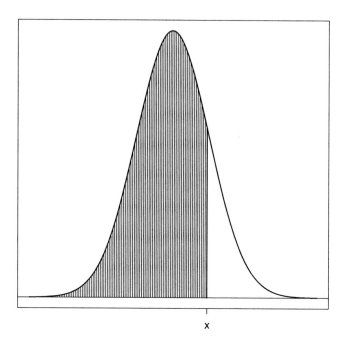

x

Figure A.1 The area under the standard normal to the left of x is given by pnorm(x) in **R**.

A.2   Chi-Squared Distribution

The **R** function pchisq provides the *lower* tail area but we are usually interested in the upper tail. The upper tail area is obtained using the following.

$$1 - \text{pchisq}(x, \text{df} = i)$$

Here is an example of the upper tail areas for $x = 1, \ldots, 5$ and df equal to 1, 2 and 3.

```
> (x <- 1:5)
[1] 1 2 3 4 5
> for (i in 1:3)
+ {
+        print(noquote(paste("    ", i, " df:")))
+        print(1 - pchisq(x, df = i))
+ }
[1]      1  df:
[1] 0.31731051 0.15729921 0.08326452 0.04550026 0.02534732
[1]      2  df:
[1] 0.6065307 0.3678794 0.2231302 0.1353353 0.0820850
[1]      3  df:
[1] 0.8012520 0.5724067 0.3916252 0.2614641 0.1717971
```

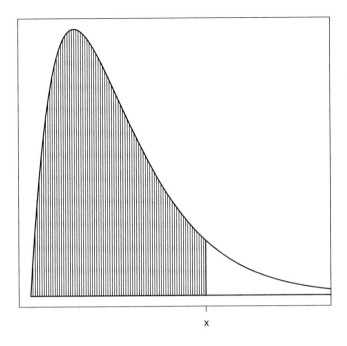

x

Figure A.2 For specified value x, the `pchisq` function provides the corresponding lower shaded area.

For a given upper tail area we can also obtain the corresponding critical value using `qchisq`. The upper tail areas of 5% and 1% for df equal to 1, 2, and 3 are obtained by writing.

```
> p <- c(.95, .99)
> for (i in 1:3)
+    print(qchisq(p, df = i))
[1] 3.841459 6.634897
[1] 5.991465 9.210340
[1] 7.814728 11.344867
```

Selected Solutions and Hints

1.5 Pink eye is an infection and can often be traced to swimming in unclean water or contact with chlorine in the water.

2.2 a. We expect 2, and the standard deviation is $8 \times 0.25 \times (1 - 0.25) = 1.225$.

 b. The probability all eight are cold-free is 0.75^8. The probability three or more have a cold is

$$Pr[3 \text{ or more}] = 1 - Pr[2 \text{ or fewer}]$$
$$= 1 - (0.25^8) - (8 \times 0.25^7 \times 0.75) - (28 \times 0.25^6 \times 0.75^2).$$

 c. Is the health status of the children independent?

2.3 a. Alternative hypotheses further away from the null hypothesis have greater power. Intuitively, it is easy to tell whether the null or alternative hypothesis is true when these are very different.

 b. The alternative furthest from the null hypothesis has the greatest power, but such alternatives are rarely useful to us. If such a large difference existed and was visible, then it would already be well known.

 c. As the sample size increases, we are able to test hypotheses closer together and more subtle differences can be detected.

2.5 The probability of a kangaroo flush, or any other five-card hand for that matter, is

$$1 \bigg/ \binom{52}{5} = \frac{5 \times 4 \times 3 \times 2 \times 1}{52 \times 51 \times 50 \times 49 \times 48} = 3.85 \times 10^{-7}.$$

2.8 c. Are the occurrences of infections independent events?

3.3 a. Two infants who differ by 1 cm in length should differ in average weight by about 61.65 g.

 b. The estimated intercept would correspond to the estimated weight of an infant with zero length.

3.6 This is a map of residuals. Notice Washington State and Texas, which respectively have large and small amounts of rain, are receiving normal amounts according to this map.

3.8 Use a t-test to compare attendance records for teams with and without playoff appearances.

4.1 The variance is not constant. It is increasing with more recent years. The residuals are also correlated: Profitable years are also followed by other profitable years. There was a large outlier (loss) in 2007.

4.2 Three points can achieve a correlation of $+1$ or -1 if they all fall on a straight line with nonzero slope.

4.3 Adding a constant to all values does not change the correlation. Neither does multiplying by a positive number. Multiplying by a negative number reverses the sign of the correlation coefficient.

4.4 The complete ANOVA is as follows.

Source	df	Sum of squares	Mean square	F value
Model	1	32.0	32.0	4.0
Error	20	160.0	8.0	
Total	21	192.0		

4.7 These are the residuals from the regression: Does there appear to be an increase in variability with estimated attendance?

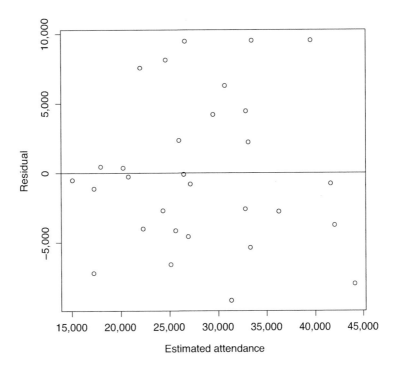

5.1 The model with as many parameters as observations will have 0 df for error. It will also have a perfect fit and $R^2 = 1$. Such a model is useless because it offers no simplification of the original data.

6.4 This is an example of regression to the mean.

6.5 The four assumptions are as follows.

1. The errors in each of the groups are independent.
2. The errors in each group have the same variances.

3. All errors in all groups have zero means.

4. The errors in each group have normal distributions.

6.6 This is the spaghetti plot resulting from plotting each country's attitudes over time.

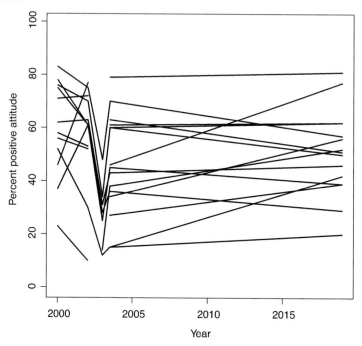

6.7 If consumption is measured on a linear scale, we have

$$\text{Price} = \alpha + \beta C,$$

where C is the per-person average daily consumption. If C increases by one unit, then the estimated price increases by β dollars.

When consumption is measured on a log scale, the model is

$$\text{Price} = \alpha + \beta \log(C).$$

If we double consumption, then

$$\text{Price} = \alpha + \beta \log(2C)$$
$$= \alpha + \beta \log(C) + \beta \log(2)$$

shows the estimated price increases by $\beta \log(2)$.

9.1 Recall $\log(x) = -\log(1/x)$. Then

$$\log\left(\frac{p}{1-p}\right) = -\log\left(\frac{1-p}{p}\right),$$

so we only have to reverse the signs of the fitted regression coefficients in the computer output.

9.4.4 If we fit a logistic regression model, the response variable is whether the record high occurs later or earlier than the record low. The explanatory variables in this model were the record minimum temperature, maximum temperature, and maximum temperature squared. Several dates in early December are influential as given in this plot of the hat matrix diagonals.

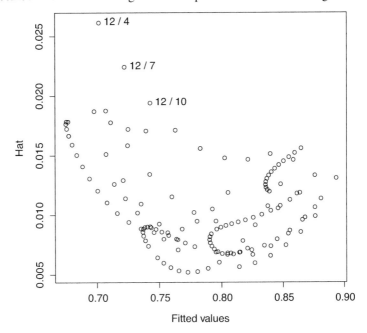

10.6.7 In general, the age effects are increasing and the cohort effects are decreasing.

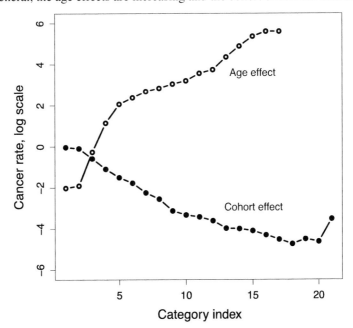

13.1 Survival analysis is appropriate. The outcome is time to recovery, defined as a certain level of ambulatory independence. Some wheelchair-bound individuals never recover and should be considered censored. We can use proportional hazards regression to model the effects of covariates such as age, sex, and the need for a home health aide. The null hypothesis is that none of these has any effect on time to recovery.

13.2 This is an example of the Poisson model. Square holes are rare, but a large number of doughnuts are produced. We can perform a Poisson regression to see if the temperature or coating resulted in different numbers of defective doughnuts. The null hypothesis is these have no effect on the number of defective doughnuts.

13.3 This is an example of survival analysis with right censoring. We know when the bill is introduced (left end point) and the day it passes (right end point) or whether it is still pending legislative approval (censored). Proportional hazards regression can be used to see if the type of bill or the party sponsoring it is useful in explaining how long it took to pass. The null hypothesis is these explanatory variables are not useful.

13.4 Linear regression might be useful here. Stopping distance is always positive but never censored. We can model the effects of pavement conditions, make and model of car, and color. The null hypothesis is none if these factors influence stopping distance.

13.5 If everybody received either an A or a B, then these binary-valued outcomes should be modeled using logistic regression. The null hypothesis is sex, age, major, and other courses have no relationship to the grade in the course.

13.6 When we learn the data has a lot of noise, we should use nonparametric methods. The rank-sum or median test can compare evaluations from required or elective course students. The null hypothesis is these should be about the same.

13.7 In this linear regression we might use 12 indicator variables – one for each month. We might also use four indicators for each of the four seasons. The null hypothesis is housing starts are the same year-round.

13.8 We might use logistic regression because the responses are either improved status or not. Because almost all patients recover, the trial is large, and the probability of failure is so small, we might also use Poisson regression. The null hypothesis in either of these regressions is that there is no difference in the failure rate for the two different drugs.

13.9 Every record is either proper or improper. These binary-valued outcomes should be modeled using logistic regression. The null hypothesis is the patient's sex, age, comorbidity, and type of health insurance have no effect on the likelihood of the an improper use of their HIPAA information.

13.10 We can use survival analysis here to model the time until relapse. Patients who have not relapsed at the time of the statistical analysis are considered censored. The null hypothesis in proportional hazards regression is that these covariates have no effect on the relapse time.

13.11 There are many people at risk for rabies, but the chances of contracting it are very small. The Poisson regression is appropriate here. The null hypothesis is that there is no trend.

13.12 This is a 2 × 2 table of frequencies. We count the number of people who are either old or young and are either cat owners or not. We might use the chi-squared or exact test to see if age is related to ownership. The null hypothesis is that these are independent of each other.

13.13 If age is measured on a continuous scale, then we should use logistic regression to model the binary-valued outcome of cat ownership or not. The null hypothesis is that age does not matter.

13.14 Every individual is either a case or a control. If tobacco use is also binary valued, then we can analyze these data using a chi-squared test for this 2 × 2 table of frequencies. The null hypothesis is that the risk of disease is not related to tobacco use. We can also use logistic regression to compare education levels in the case-control data. The null hypothesis is that education level is independent of the risk of disease.

13.15 The linear logistic model of the probability P of dying is

$$\text{logit}(P) = \alpha + \beta \, \text{Dose}, \qquad (S.1)$$

where

$$\text{logit}(P) = \log \left(\frac{P}{1 - P} \right).$$

a. The null hypothesis is $\beta = 0$, and the alternative is β is different from zero.

b. When $P = 0.5$, then

$$\text{logit}(P) = \log(0.5/0.5) = \log(1) = 0.$$

If $\alpha = -3$ and $\beta = 0.5$, then solving for Dose in (S.1) gives us Dose $= 6$ as the estimated LD_{50}.

13.35 The survival curve goes all the way to zero if the longest-surviving individual has his or her event. The survival curve will stop before reaching zero if the longest-surviving individual is censored.

13.37 Unreliable data with known outliers such as these are good candidates for nonparametric methods.

References

Abbruzzese JL, Madden T, Sugarman SM, *et al.* (1996). Phase I clinical and plasma and cellular pharmacological study of topotecan with and without granulocyte colony-stimulating factor. *Clinical Cancer Research* **2**: 1489–97.

Andrews DF and Herzberg AM (1985). *Data.* New York: Springer-Verlag.

Anscombe FJ (1973). Graphs in statistical analysis, *American Statistician* **27**: 17–21.

Cokol M, Chua HN, Tasan M, *et al.* (2011). Systematic exploration of synergistic drug pairs. *Molecular Systems Biology* **7**: Article number 544; https://doi.org/10.1038/msb.2011.71

Cox DR (1972). Regression models and life-tables. *Journal of the Royal Statistical Society. Series B (Methodological)* **34**(2): 187–220.

Dobson AJ (2002). *An Introduction to Generalized Linear Models*, second edition. Boca Raton, FL: Chapman & Hall.

Efron B (1978). Regression and ANOVA with zero-one data: Measures of residual variation. *Journal of the American Statistical Association* **73**: 113–21.

Embury SH, Elias L, Heller PH, *et al.* (1977). Remission maintenance therapy in acute myclogenous leukemia. *Western Journal of Medicine* **126**: 267–72.

Farmer JH, Kodell RL, Greenman DL, and Shaw GW (1979). Dose and time response models for the incidence of bladder and liver neoplasms in mice fed 2-acetylaminofluorene continuously. *Journal of Environmental Pathology and Toxicology* **3**: 55–68.

Fleming T, O'Fallon JR, O'Brien PD, and Harrington DP (1980). Modified Kolmogorov–Smirnov test procedures with application to arbitrarily right-censored data. *Biometrics* **36**: 607–25.

Friedland L, Joffe M, Moore D, *et al.* (1992). Effect of educational program on compliance with glove use in a pediatric emergency department. *American Journal of Diseases of Childhood* **146**: 1355–8.

Frisby JP and Clatworthy, JL (1975). Learning to see complex random-dot stereograms. *Perception* **4**: 173–8.

Glovsky L and Rigrodsky S (1964). A developmental analysis of mentally deficient children with early histories of aphasis. *Training School Bulletin* **61**: 76–96.

Hart J (2015). Association between air temperature and cancer death rates in Florida: An ecological study *Dose Response* **13**(1); https://doi.org/10.2203/dose-response.14-024.Hart.

Innes JRM, Ulland BM, Valerio MG, *et al.* (1969). Bioassay of pesticides and industrial chemicals for tumorigenicity in mice: A preliminary note. *Journal of the National Cancer Institute* **42**: 1101–14.

Kannisto V (1988). On the survival of centenarians and the span of life. *Population Studies* **42**: 389–406.

Kaplan EL and Meier P (1958). Nonparametric estimation from incomplete observations. *Journal of the American Statistical Association* **53**: 457–81.

Koziol JA, Maxwell DA, Fukushima M, Colmerauer MEM, and Pilch YH (1981). A distribution-free test for tumor-growth curve analysis with application to an animal tumor immunotherapy experiment. *Biometrics* **37**: 383–90.

Lange N, Ryan L, Billard L, *et al.* (editors) (1984). *Case Studies in Biometry.* New York: Wiley.

Lea AJ (1965). New observations on distribution of neoplasms of female breast in certain European countries. *British Medical Journal* **1**(5433): 488–90.

Lee JAH, Hitosugi M, and Peterson GR (1973). Rise in mortality from tumors of the testis in Japan, 1947–70. *Journal of the National Cancer Institute* **51**: 1485–90.

Mackenzie CA, Lockridge A, and Keith M. (2005). Declining sex ratio in a first nation community. *Environmental Health Perspectives* **113**: 1295–8.

Mosteller F and Tukey JW (1977). *Data Analysis and Regression. A Second Course in Statistics.* Reading, MA: Addison-Wesley.

Pagano M and Gauvreau K (2000). *Principles of Biostatistics*, second edition. Pacific Grove, CA: Duxbury.

Plackett RL (1981). *The Analysis of Categorical Data*, second edition. London: Charles Griffin.

Remington JS, Efron B, Cavanaugh E, Simon HJ, and Trejos A (1970). Studies on toxoplasmosis in El Salvador. Prevalence and incidence of toxoplasmosis as measured by the Sabin-Feldman dye test. *Transactions of the Royal Society of Tropical Medicine and Hygiene* **64**: 252–67; https://doi.org/10.1016/0035-9203(70)90132-x. PMID: 5449051.

Rose CS, Nielsen JK, Gauvin JR, *et al.* (2019). Survival outcome patterns revealed by deploying advanced tags in quantity: Pacific halibut (*Hippoglossus stenolepis*) survivals after release from trawl catches through expedited sorting (2019). *Canadian Journal of Fisheries and Aquatic Sciences* **76**: 2215-24; https://doi.org/10.1139/cjfas-2018-0350.

Smith D and Von Behren J (2005). Trends in the sex ratio of California births, 1960–1996. *Journal of Epidemiology and Community Health* **59**: 1047–53.

Stuckler D, King LP, and Basu S (2008). International Monetary Fund programs and tuberculosis outcomes in post-communist countries *PLOS Medicine*. Available online at https://doi.org/10.1371/journal.pmed.0050143.

Teasdale N, Bard C, LaRue J, and Fleury M (1993). On the cognitive penetrability of posture control. *Experimental Aging Research* **19**: 1–13.

Tufte ER (2011). *The Visual Display of Quantitative Information*, second edition. Cheshire, CT: Graphics Press.

van Wattum PJ, Chappell PB, Zelterman D, Scahill LD, and Lecktman JF (2000). Patterns of response to acute naxolone infusion in Tourette's syndrome. *Movement Disorders* **15**: 1252–4.

Wheler J, Tsimberidou AM, Hong D, *et al.* (2009). Survival of patients in a Phase I clinic. *Cancer* **115**: 1091–9.

Wilkinson L (2005). *The Grammar of Graphics*, second edition. New York: Springer.

Zelterman D (1992). A statistical distribution with an unbounded hazard function and its application to a theory from demography. *Biometrics* **48**: 807–18.

Index